Applied Communicable Disease Control

Understanding Public Health Series

Series editors: Nicki Thorogood and Rosalind Plowman, London School of Hygiene & Tropical Medicine

Throughout the world, recognition of the importance of public health to sustainable, safe, and healthy societies is growing. The achievements of public health in nineteenth-century Europe were for much of the twentieth century overshadowed by advances in personal care, in particular in-hospital care. Now, with the dawning of a new century, there is increasing understanding of the inevitable limits of individual health care and of the need to complement such services with effective public health strategies. Major improvements in people's health will come from controlling communicable diseases, eradicating environmental hazards, improving people's diets, and enhancing the availability and quality of effective health care. To achieve this, every country needs a cadre of knowledgeable public health practitioners with social, political, and organizational skills to lead and bring about changes at international, national, and local levels.

This is one of a series of books that provides a foundation for those wishing to join in and contribute to the twenty-first-century regeneration of public health, helping to put the concerns and perspectives of public health at the heart of policy-making and service provision. While each book stands alone, together they provide a comprehensive account of the three main aims of public health: protecting the public from environmental hazards, improving the health of the public, and ensuring high-quality health services are available to all. Some of the books focus on methods, others on key topics. They have been written by staff at the London School of Hygiene & Tropical Medicine with considerable experience of teaching public health to students from low-, middle-, and high-income countries. Much of the material has been developed and tested with postgraduate students both in face-to-face teaching and through distance learning.

The books are designed for self-directed learning. In each chapter, there are explicit learning objectives, highlighted key terms, and many activities to enable the reader to test their own understanding of the ideas and material covered. Written in a clear and accessible style, the series will be essential reading for students taking postgraduate courses in public health and will also be of interest to public health practitioners and policy-makers.

Titles in the series

Analytical models for decision making: Colin Sanderson and Reinhold Gruen
Applied communicable disease control: Liza Cragg, Will Nutland and James Rudge (eds.)
Conflict and health: Natasha Howard, Egbert Sondorp, and Annemarie Ter Veen (eds.)
Controlling communicable disease: Norman Noah
Economic analysis for management and policy: Stephen Jan, Lilani Kumaranayake, Jenny Roberts, Kara Hanson, and Kate Archibald
Economic evaluation: Julia Fox-Rushby and John Cairns (eds.)
Environmental epidemiology: Paul Wilkinson (ed.)
Environmental health policy: Megan Landon and Tony Fletcher
Environment, health and sustainable development, Second Edition: Emma Hutchinson and Sari Kovats
Financial management in health services: Reinhold Gruen and Anne Howarth
Health care evaluation, Second Edition: Carmen Tsang and David Cromwell
Health promotion theory, Second Edition: Liza Cragg, Maggie Davies, and Wendy MacDowall (eds.)
Health promotion practice, Second Edition: Will Nutland and Liza Cragg (eds.)
Introduction to epidemiology, Third Edition: Ilona Carneiro
Introduction to health economics, Second Edition: Lorna Guinness and Virginia Wiseman (eds.)
Issues in public health, Second Edition: Fiona Sim and Martin McKee (eds.)
Making health policy, Second Edition: Kent Buse, Nicholas Mays, and Gill Walt
Managing health services: Nick Goodwin, Reinhold Gruen, and Valerie Iles
Medical anthropology: Robert Pool and Wenzel Geissler
Principles of social research, Second Edition: Mary Alison Durand and Tracey Chantler (eds.)
Public health in history: Virginia Berridge, Martin Gorsky, and Alex Mold
Sexual health: *A public health perspective*: Kay Wellings, Kirstin Mitchell, and Martine Collumbien (eds.)
Understanding health services, Second Edition: Ipek Gürol-Urgancı, Fiona Campbell, and Nick Black

Applied Communicable Disease Control

Liza Cragg, Will Nutland and James Rudge

Open University Press

Open University Press
McGraw-Hill Education
8th Floor, 338 Euston Road
London
England
NW1 3BH

and Two Penn Plaza, New York, NY 10121-2289, USA

First published 2018

Commissioning Editor: Vivien Antwi
Development Editor: Tom Payne
Editorial Assistant: Karen Harris
Content Product Manager: Ali Davis

A catalogue record of this book is available from the British Library

ISBN-13: 9780335262922
ISBN-10: 0335262929
eISBN: 9780335262939

Library of Congress Cataloging-in-Publication Data
CIP data applied for

Typeset by Transforma Pvt. Ltd., Chennai, India

Printed and bound in Great Britain by Bell and Bain Ltd, Glasgow

Fictitious names of companies, products, people, characters and/or data that may be used herein (in case studies or in examples) are not intended to represent any real individual, company, product or event.

Contents

List of figures and tables

Figures

Tables

List of editors and contributors

SAMUEL BOLAND is a PhD candidate in Public Health and Policy at the London School of Hygiene & Tropical Medicine, currently focusing on the application of military and security apparatus to public health crises.

LIZA CRAGG is a freelance consultant specializing in international health who teaches on several public health distance learning modules at the London School of Hygiene & Tropical Medicine.

WILL NUTLAND is a freelance consultant specializing in HIV prevention and sexual health, and is an Honorary Assistant Professor at the London School of Hygiene & Tropical Medicine. He was formerly head of health promotion at the UK's Terrence Higgins Trust and a public health strategist for the London Borough of Tower Hamlets.

JAMES RUDGE is Assistant Professor of Infectious Disease Epidemiology at the London School of Hygiene & Tropical Medicine. Based overseas in Southeast Asia, his research focuses on understanding disease transmission dynamics at the human–animal interface to inform 'One Health'-related surveillance and control strategies.

Acknowledgements

This book builds on the face-to-face *Applied Communicable Disease Control* module and the previous distance learning module *Communicable Disease Control*, which are taught as part of the Master's in Public Health at the London School of Hygiene & Tropical Medicine. These modules have evolved over several years under the influence of many staff. The authors are grateful to all these staff for providing learning materials and ideas that have been incorporated into this book. In particular, we would like to thank Sue Cliffe, Malwina Carrion, Ros Plowman and Nicki Thorogood for their advice on the structure and content of this edition. We would also like to thank organizations and individuals who granted permission for material to be used in this book.

Overview of the book

For much of human history, communicable diseases have been a major cause of mortality and morbidity. Frequent epidemics of diseases such as small-pox, bubonic plague, cholera and typhus could rapidly kill many thousands of people. Before the causes of communicable disease were understood, efforts to prevent and to control epidemics remained ineffective. The nineteenth and twentieth centuries saw major scientific developments that led to accurate understanding of the causes of communicable disease and increasingly effective prevention and treatment. Breakthroughs including the development of vaccination and the discovery of antibiotics dramatically reduced mortality from communicable disease and led to increases in life expectancy in indus-trialized countries in the nineteenth and twentieth centuries. By the 1950s, this led some scientists to believe that communicable disease would be successfully conquered (Spellberg and Taylor-Blake, 2013).

However, since then it has become clear that communicable diseases, far from passing into history, continue to be a major threat to human health. New communicable diseases such as HIV/AIDS and Ebola virus disease (EVD) have emerged with devastating consequences. In addition, other well-known diseases, such as malaria and tuberculosis (TB), have proven much more dif-ficult to control than anticipated and continue to cause considerable mortality. Poverty and lack of access to essential health services, including vaccina-tion, continue to result in millions of preventable deaths every year from communicable disease in low-income countries. In low-income countries, communicable diseases such as lower respiratory infections, HIV/AIDS, diarrhoeal diseases, malaria and TB combined account for almost one-third of all deaths (WHO, 2017).

Why study communicable disease control?

Although communicable disease continues to present a threat to human health, there are a range of measures that can be used to reduce the harm it causes. *Communicable disease control* is the process of intervening to reduce disease incidence, prevalence, morbidity or mortality. It forms an important part of public health practice. Control measures include surveil-lance, vaccination, prevention and outbreak response.

As this book makes clear, controlling communicable disease is far from straightforward. There are many communicable diseases, which have differ-ent causes and are transmitted in different ways. Applying control measures effectively requires a good understanding of the causes of communicable disease, including the complex interaction of environmental factors, individual and population group risk factors, and the characteristics of the specific disease-causing agent.

Marginalized groups may have increased vulnerability to communicable disease and find it difficult to access health services. In certain situations, poorly designed communicable disease control strategies risk further marginalizing some groups. This book explains how to design and apply communicable disease control to address the needs of marginalized groups.

Communicable disease control strategies must be carefully designed, planned, managed and implemented in order to be effective and cost-efficient. The follow-up and evaluation of interventions also needs to ensure that, where possible, they generate learning which can contribute to developing the evidence base of what works. Careful consideration needs to be given to the ethical implications of action to control communicable disease. Attention is also needed to ensure communication with the public does not lead to fear, which is counterproductive to control.

This book is designed to provide readers with an overview of communicable disease control measures and the knowledge and skills to apply these in different contexts and for diverse populations.

The structure of the book

This book is structured in three sections. The first of these sections, which is made up of three chapters, explains the causes of communicable disease. The second section, which comprises four chapters, looks at the range of different measures that are used to control communicable disease. The third section, which consists of four chapters, explores how to apply these measures.

Each chapter follows the same format. A brief overview tells you about the contents, followed by learning objectives and the key terms you will encounter. There are several activities in each chapter, which are designed to help you apply the learning and tools introduced in the chapter and to test knowledge and understanding. Each activity is followed by feedback to enable you to check on your own understanding. If things are not clear, then you are encouraged to go back and re-read the material.

Section 1: Understanding communicable disease

Chapter 1 provides a brief historical introduction to communicable disease. It describes how the causes of communicable disease were understood historically and how this understanding developed. The chapter also explores how early efforts to control communicable disease evolved, including the key components of communicable disease control in use today. The chapter then briefly discusses how improvements in communicable disease control have impacted health outcomes.

Chapter 2 explores the factors that contribute to causing communicable diseases. It introduces the epidemiologic triad, a model that conceptualizes communicable disease causation as an interaction of factors relating to agent, host and environment. It then describes the different types of agents that can cause communicable disease and the factors that influence whether a person develops a disease.

Chapter 3 explains the chain of infection whereby an infectious agent enters a susceptible host and the places where infectious agents live and multiply, known as reservoirs. It then explains the different ways an infectious agent can enter a susceptible host, which are known as modes of transmission.

These first three chapters enable the reader to develop an understanding of how communicable disease is transmitted, which is an important step in developing effective measures to control it.

Section 2: Measures to control communicable disease

The second section of this book turns to the measures that are used to control communicable disease. Chapter 4 explains the crucial role surveillance plays in controlling communicable disease, exploring what surveillance is and what it is used for. It describes the overall design of a surveillance system, the activities that make up communicable disease surveillance, including the types of data that are used, and the essential features of a communicable disease surveillance system.

Chapter 5 explains how vaccination is used to prevent and control communicable disease, including how vaccination works and the types of vaccine currently available. It describes the main strategies used to design and deliver vaccination programmes, and explores practical considerations for their success and some of the challenges involved.

Chapter 6 addresses the strategies that can be used to prevent outbreaks of communicable disease in addition to vaccination. These strategies include reducing exposure and the risk of transmission, reducing the number of contacts infected people have with others, reducing the infectious period and eradicating the disease. The chapter also describes the actions that are commonly used in each of these strategies, including action to address the causes of communicable disease and support capacity for effective prevention.

Chapter 7 explores how communicable disease control measures, including surveillance, prevention and vaccination, are applied in the event of an outbreak. The chapter describes what outbreaks are and why they occur. It explains why it is important to respond to outbreaks, who the key players in outbreak response are and the key stages of outbreak response.

Section 3: Application of measures to control communicable disease

The final section of the book discusses how the measures explained in Section 2 can be applied in practice. Chapter 8 explains how communication is at the heart of any communicable disease control strategy. It highlights the role of mass and social media and introduces some of the most commonly used methods of communication, such as press releases, press conferences, media interviews, case studies and communication outreach to key communities. The chapter explains some of the key features of effective communication, including some of the commonly used techniques for communicating uncertainty and risk.

Chapter 9 explores the ethics of communicable disease control and introduces ethical frameworks that can be used to evaluate communicable disease control strategies. It explores the fundamental principles of ethics, including those specifically for public health practice and the application of communicable disease control. The chapter includes an analysis of how responses to communicable disease control can be driven by fear, and the ethical consequences of fear-driven approaches.

Chapter 10 describes health systems, highly complex structures that exist both formally and informally, and the crucial role they play in communicable disease control. The chapter describes different types of health system and models of health care, including resource availability and evidence-based practice. It then explores current health system trends.

The final chapter, Chapter 11, explores emerging trends in communicable disease and the environmental, economic and social factors that are driving these trends. The chapter examines antimicrobial resistance, one of the key challenges to communicable disease control, and explores developments in global health governance and financing and critiques of these. It concludes by outlining developing opportunities for communicable disease control.

Brief explanation of terminology

There are several terms that are used in public health practice and research literature to describe diseases that spread between people. In particular, the terms 'communicable', 'infectious' and 'contagious' are often used synonymously. An infectious disease is a disease caused by the entrance into the body of organisms that grow and multiply there. A communicable disease is an infectious disease transmissible by direct contact with an affected individual or the individual's discharges or by indirect means through a vector. As some infectious diseases are not spread from person to person, not all infectious diseases are communicable diseases. However, because the vast majority of infectious diseases are communicable, the two terms tend to be used interchangeably. This book adopts this practice. A contagious disease is an infectious disease transmitted by person to person. This does not include diseases that can only be transmitted by vectors. However, the term 'contagious disease' is sometimes used as a synonym for infectious disease. To avoid confusion, this book does not use the term 'contagious disease'. Chapter 1 discusses these terms in more detail.

Each chapter includes a list of key terms used in that chapter and their definitions in its opening paragraphs. These key terms are brought together in a glossary at the end of the book.

References

Spellberg, B. and Taylor-Blake, B. (2013) On the exoneration of Dr. William H. Stewart: debunking an urban legend, *Infectious Diseases of Poverty*, 2 (1): 3.

World Health Organization (WHO) (2017) *The top 10 causes of death*, Fact Sheet. Available at: http://www.who.int/mediacentre/factsheets/fs310/en/index2.html

SECTION 1

Understanding communicable disease

A brief history of the development of communicable disease control

Liza Cragg

Overview

This chapter provides a brief historical introduction to communicable disease. It describes how the causes of communicable disease were understood historically and how this understanding developed, culminating in germ theory. The chapter also explores how early efforts to control communicable disease developed, including the evolution of the key components of communicable disease control in use today. Finally, the chapter briefly discusses how improvements in communicable disease control have impacted health outcomes.

Learning objectives

After reading this chapter, you will be able to:

- describe important developments in the understanding of the causes of communicable diseases
- describe how key communicable disease control activities developed
- understand the impact on health outcomes of these developments over time

Key terms

Bacterium: The singular of bacteria.

Communicable disease: An infectious disease transmissible by direct contact with an affected individual or the individual's discharges, or by indirect means through a vector (see Box 1.1).

Disease: An abnormal condition that has signs and symptoms, which may affect the whole body or any of its parts.

Disease control: In this context, the reduction of disease incidence, prevalence, morbidity or mortality to a locally acceptable level as a result of deliberate efforts (Dowdle and Cochi, 2011).

Disease elimination: The reduction to zero of the incidence of a specified disease in a defined geographical area as a result of deliberate efforts.

Disease eradication: The permanent reduction to zero of the worldwide incidence of infection of that disease as a result of deliberate efforts.

Horizontal disease control: Disease control programmes that are integrated into and delivered as a part of the provision of general health services to the population.

Immunization: The process whereby a person is made immune or resistant to an infectious disease, typically by the administration of a vaccine.

Infectious disease: A disease caused by the entrance into the body of infectious agents that grow and multiply there (see Box 1.1).

Vertical disease control: Disease control programmes that are concerned with specific health conditions and problems.

Communicable disease in history

Communicable diseases are likely to have been present in some form throughout human history. However, research indicates that most of the communicable diseases known today have emerged within the past 11,000 years, after the development of agriculture (Wolfe et al., 2007). There are a number of reasons for this. First, infectious diseases of humans can only be sustained where there are large numbers of human beings living together in dense conditions. These conditions came into being as a result of the population explosion that followed the introduction of agriculture. The hunter-gatherer societies that preceded agriculture were not sufficiently populous and concentrated to allow the development and spread of infectious diseases. Second, after the introduction of agriculture people began to travel more, facilitating wider geographic spread. Third, people had much closer contact with animals as a result of agriculture and these animals had pathogens, which, over time, transformed into pathogens causing infectious diseases in humans (Jones, 2016).

Box 1.1: Communicable, infectious or contagious?

An infectious disease is a disease caused by the entrance into the body of organisms that grow and multiply there. A communicable disease is an infectious disease transmissible by direct contact with an affected individual or the individual's discharges or by indirect means through a vector (Merriam-Webster, 2016). The word 'communicable' refers to the fact that the disease can be communicated, or transmitted, from one person to another. As some infectious diseases are not spread from person to person, not all infectious diseases are communicable diseases. For example, tetanus is a non-communicable disease caused by the bacterium *Clostridium tetani* (WHO, 2016a). However, because the vast majority of infectious diseases are communicable, the two terms tend to be used interchangeably. This book adopts this practice. A contagious disease is an infectious disease transmitted by person-to-person contact. This does not include diseases that can only be transmitted by vectors. However, the term contagious disease is sometimes used as a synonym for infectious disease. To avoid confusion, this book does not use the term contagious disease.

The earliest evidence of the existence of infectious diseases comes from ancient history. For example, human skeletal remains indicate that lepromatous leprosy, the most serious form of leprosy that affects the skin, nerves and other organs, was present in India in 2000 BCE (Robbins *et al.*, 2009) and tuberculosis (TB) bacteria have been found in ancient human skeletal remains from the Neolithic period (Hershkovitz *et al.*, 2008). Human remains, carvings and manuscripts from ancient Egypt indicate that specific diseases, including TB, malaria, polio and smallpox, were present there (see, for example, Figure 1.1). Furthermore, written accounts from ancient history document epidemics with very high mortality rates from diseases that cannot be identified with certainty; examples include the outbreak known as 'the Plague of Athens' in 430 BCE and 'the Antonine Plague' of 165–180 CE in Rome. The first major outbreak of the bubonic plague occurred in the Byzantine Empire, beginning in 542 CE, and resulted in an estimated 25 million deaths. A second major outbreak of the bubonic plague occurred in Europe between 1347 and 1351, where it was known as the Black Death, and killed 25–50% of Europe's population (Gottfried, 2010).

Early efforts to control communicable diseases

Up until the second half of the nineteenth century when Robert Koch, building on the work of earlier scientists, described a coherent theory of germs, physicians and scientists based explanations for the occurrence of diseases on

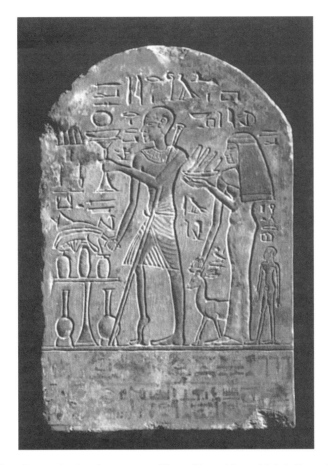

Figure 1.1 An Egyptian stele showing a man with a withered leg which is thought to represent a person with polio. 18th Dynasty (1403–1365 BC). The stele is in the collection of the Glyptoteket museum

superstition, religion and primitive environmental theories such as bad air (known as 'miasma'). Early efforts to control the spread of infection were based on observation of patients. From this, scientists and physicians had understood there was a relationship between getting a disease and being close to or in contact with an infected person. However, because the existence of microorganisms and their role in causing infectious disease was not understood, efforts to control their spread were largely ineffective. This section explores important developments in early efforts to control communicable disease.

Quarantine

One early effort to control the spread of infectious disease was through quarantine. Quarantine refers to the practice of separating and restricting

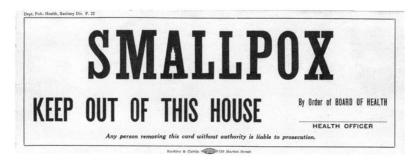

Figure 1.2 A Board of Health quarantine poster dating from the early twentieth century in San Francisco, California

Source: Copyright © Public Domain. By San Francisco, California: Buckley & Curtin, [191-]. Courtesy of the National Library of Medicine. Images from the History of Medicine (IHM), http://resource.nlm.nih.gov/101392841. HMD Prints & Photos call number: WA 234 C25 no. 14 sol.

the movement of people who have been exposed to a contagious disease to see if they become sick. The word quarantine stems from the Italian word *quaranta*, or 'forty', which refers to the forty days of enforced isolation that arriving ships were subjected to before being allowed entry to Venice (Mackowiak and Sehdev, 2002). This practice was introduced in the fourteenth century, at the height of the outbreak of the Black Death. While crude in design, early Venetian public health practitioners recognized that the disease was arriving from abroad. They believed if they could observe new arrivals for a period of time to see if they developed symptoms and prevent them from entering if they did, they would be able to protect the city from the disease. As well as being used against bubonic plague, quarantine was enlisted in Europe and the Americas from the seventeenth century against smallpox, cholera, TB and influenza (Tognotti, 2013). For example, Figure 1.2 shows a poster dating from the early twentieth century in San Francisco, California where quarantine was used for an outbreak of smallpox.

Epidemiology

John Snow, a British physician in the nineteenth century, contributed significantly to the development of epidemiology, which has since become an essential component of communicable disease control. The first significant cholera outbreak in London took place in 1832, with more outbreaks in the years that followed. At that time, most clinicians thought cholera was caused by atmospheric 'effluence' or 'miasma'. In 1854, a cholera outbreak in the Soho area of London caused significant mortality. Based on his earlier observations of cholera, Snow was sceptical about the theory that the cause was 'effluence' or 'miasma'. By systematically interviewing people affected in the outbreak and mapping the addresses of those who died, Snow was able to determine the exposures that those affected had in common. This led him to suspect a water pump on Broad Street was the source of the outbreak. He intervened to ensure the local council removed the pump handle, thus preventing people from drawing water from the well (Cameron and Jones, 1983). Because of Snow's systematic approach, the speed of his action, the logic of his analysis and the response it led to, this event is considered an important milestone in the development of epidemiology and its use in communicable disease control.

Hygiene

The World Health Organization (WHO) defines hygiene as 'conditions and practices that help to maintain health and prevent the spread of diseases' (WHO, 2016b). Practices around hygiene have existed for many centuries. Some ancient civilizations are known to have had well-developed sanitation infrastructure. For example, in ancient Crete, efforts to address hygiene in populated areas date back to 3000 BCE when large-scale sewage treatment facilities to remove contaminated water out to sea were introduced (Angelakis *et al.*, 2014). Ancient Romans understood the importance of the provision of clean water for health and built an extensive system of aqueducts to ensure its supply. However, according to historical sources, access to clean water in medieval Europe was inadequate and hygiene practices were in general poor (Amulree, 1973).

Over the course of the nineteenth century, the population of Western European nations grew rapidly. This population growth was accompanied by industrialization and urbanization. Living and working conditions in the rapidly expanding cities were extremely poor and infectious diseases, including cholera and typhoid, thrived. From the 1830s onwards, prominent members of society, scientists, physicians and journalists in Britain advocated for improvements by writing to newspapers, contributing funds and undertaking independent research. Edwin Chadwick was a key figure in the campaign for sanitary reform in Britain, which became known as the British Sanitary Movement and laid the foundations for the development of public health. In 1848, Chadwick oversaw the introduction of the Public Health Act. By the second half of the nineteenth century, sanitarian reform in Britain, including the removal of refuse, the construction of sewage systems and the provision of clean water, was well underway (Hamlin, 1998).

Medical hygiene, the practices used in the prevention of infections during medical treatment, developed in the nineteenth and twentieth centuries. One of the pioneers of infection control in hospitals was Ignaz Semmelweis. In 1847, based in part on his observations of the incidence of puerperal fever in different settings, Semmelweis recommended hand washing prior to assisting with childbirth and subsequently observed the incidence of puerperal fever decline significantly where hand washing was adopted. Florence Nightingale, who is often credited as the founder of modern nursing as a profession, also contributed to the development of hospital hygiene practices.

Public health

Public health can be defined as 'the art and science of preventing disease, prolonging life and promoting health through the organized efforts of society' (Acheson, 1988). As discussed earlier, public health as a discipline developed from the British Sanitary Movement, which campaigned for improvements in water and sanitation infrastructure in cities that, as a result of industrialization in the first half of the nineteenth century, were expanding rapidly. In the late nineteenth and early twentieth century, the discipline of public health developed alongside that of clinical medicine. Whereas clinical medicine was seen to be concerned with the health of individuals, public health was concerned with the health of communities and populations. Initially, public health focused on measures to reduce epidemics of diseases that were seen as posing a threat to the political, social and economic wellbeing of the nation. Early public health policies were intended to secure the health of a working population. They often included compulsory requirements, such as obligatory vaccination against smallpox and notification of sexually transmitted diseases. For this reason, some historians have seen public health in this period as a form of social control (Donajgrodzki, 1977).

In the early twentieth century, as public health in Britain developed, it began to address the causal factors underlying public health problems, and during the 1930s and 1940s the concept of social medicine developed, which was concerned with what John Ryle described as the 'whole economic, nutritional, occupational, educational and psychological opportunity or experience of the individual or community' (Ryle, 1948: 11–12). Public health professionals inspired by social medicine began to work with local communities themselves to improve health. The 1970s saw the emergence of the new public health movement, which addressed risk, safety, prevention and individual behaviour as both a cause of and a way to reduce disease. A series of initiatives introduced by the WHO in the late 1970s and 1980s stressed the importance of promoting good health as well as combating disease. The 1978 Alma Ata Declaration, for example, advocated a multidimensional approach to health and socio-economic development, and urged active community participation in health care and health education at every level, with a particular focus on primary health care.

Immunization and vaccines

Arguably, one of the greatest developments in public health and infectious disease prevention was the introduction of immunization. The concept behind immunization is simple: limited exposure to a pathogen, or a part of a pathogen, will stimulate a person's immune system to identify and respond to that pathogen if exposed to it in the future, thereby giving immunity from infection. The practice of exposing a person to a pathogen to develop protective immunity is thought to have been used for the first time in sixteenth-century China, where it was undertaken to prevent smallpox (Deng, 2011). The procedure, known as variolation, involved rubbing powdered scabs or fluids from small-pox pustules into superficial wounds in an uninfected person. The individual would usually develop a mild form of disease localized to the site of infection and recover, having gained protective immunity against the virus. The practice spread to Europe in the early eighteenth century and became established as a medical practice in England (Dinc and Ulman, 2007). Variolation is a crude form of immunization, which carries significant risks for the recipient.

In the late eighteenth century, Edward Jenner refined the practice of vari-olation, using cowpox instead of smallpox. Cowpox is milder than smallpox in humans, but similar enough that the body develops some immunity against smallpox. Jenner had observed that typically the milkmaids of the time did not contract smallpox, as they were exposed occupationally to cowpox. He tested this theory by introducing cowpox into the arm of a young boy, who became mildly ill for 10 days and then demonstrated immunity from smallpox. Jenner called this new procedure 'vaccination', which comes from *vaccinia*, Latin for cowpox (Riedel, 2005).

In the second half of the nineteenth century, Louis Pasteur made further significant breakthroughs in the development of vaccines. Pasteur pioneered the use of an artificially generated weakened form of the disease-causing pathogen for use as a vaccine. Pasteur played a key role in the develop-ment of vaccines for anthrax and rabies.

According to the WHO there are now 25 vaccine-preventable infections. Immunization has resulted in the eradication of smallpox, lowered the global incidence of polio by 99% and reduced illness, disability and death from diphtheria, tetanus, whooping cough, measles, *Haemophilus influenzae* type b disease and epidemic meningococcal A meningitis. It has been called 'one of the most successful and cost-effective health interventions known' (WHO, 2013). Researchers are actively looking for new vaccines to provide protection against serious infections, such as human immunodeficiency virus (HIV) and Ebola. However, as discussed in Chapter 5 of this book, the challenge is not just in developing new vaccines, but in ensuring their access and uptake across populations.

Germ theory

The germ theory of disease states that many diseases are caused by the presence and action of microscopic organisms in the body. The theory was developed and accepted in the latter part of the nineteenth century by scientists in Europe. While scientists in earlier centuries had hypothesized about the existence of tiny organic materials with the capacity to spread disease, it was Robert Koch who first proposed four basic criteria for demon-strating, in a scientifically sound manner, that a disease is caused by a particular microorganism. In doing so he built on the pioneering work of other scientists, including Ignaz Semmelweis, John Snow and Louis Pasteur.

The criteria he proposed, known as Koch's postulates, are as follows:

- The microorganism must be found in abundance in all organisms suffering from the disease, but not in healthy organisms.
- The microorganism must be isolated from the diseased organism and grown in pure culture.
- The cultured microorganism should cause disease when introduced into a healthy organism.
- The microorganism must be isolated from the inoculated host and be identical to the original causative microorganism (Lederberg, 2000).

The development of germ theory marked the beginning of what has been called the 'Golden Era' of medical bacteriology. Between 1877 and 1906, it had led to the identification of twenty of the most important disease-causing microorganisms, including typhus, tetanus and TB, cholera, diphtheria and plague (Blevins and Bronze, 2010).

Antibiotics

The name antibiotic comes from the Latin *anti* (against) and the Greek *bio* (life). Antibiotics are designed to be pharmaceutical 'killing machines', capable of targeting a wide variety of bacteria. They need to be effective against targeted bacteria, while ensuring that the side-effects do not make the drug unacceptable. The antibiotic era has roots dating as far back as ancient Egypt and Greece when it was observed that certain fungi, namely moulds, were effective in treating infections (Nwaozuzu and Ebi, 2014). Patients were given mould extracts as a therapy for a variety of illnesses, including bacterial infections. Although the ancient Greeks and Egyptians did not understand this process as germ theory, they had recognized a treatment that would revolutionize communicable disease control and medicine centuries later.

In 1907, Selman Waksman discovered a chemical compound, arsphenamine, which was toxic to the bacterium that causes syphilis (Greenwood, 2007). The drug was extremely difficult to administer and was highly toxic, often resulting in serious organ damage and even death. Some years later, Alexander Fleming, a British physician and researcher working principally in the first half of the twentieth century, discovered the effectiveness of penicillin mould against bacteria by accident (Ligon, 2004). He noticed that the bacteria surrounding where the mould had landed on his plate were dead. Fleming attempted to grow the mould and further his experiments, but had difficulty in reproducing the fungus. In 1938, Howard Florey and Ernst Chain, two researchers from Oxford in the UK, continued with Fleming's experiments and found that penicillin was effective against a bacterial infection in mice. In 1941, the first human patients were treated successfully with penicillin. However, producing sufficient quantities of penicillin to

treat patients in significant numbers was very challenging. Florey travelled
to the USA to interest pharmaceutical companies in producing the drug. As
a result of the US government's recognition that penicillin could play an
important role in treating soldiers injured in the Second World War, research
into production methods was accelerated. Scientists from government,
industry and academia collaborated and, as a result, penicillin was transformed from a laboratory curiosity into a mass-produced drug in just a few
years. The collaboration to produce penicillin has been cited as an important example of how prioritizing scientific rather than economic goals can
lead to pharmaceutical breakthroughs (Quinn, 2013).

The introduction of penicillin is considered one of the most important scientific discoveries of all time. It transformed modern medicine by enabling
the successful treatment of wound infections that would previously have
proven fatal. It also enabled the control of many infectious diseases and
made surgical procedures much less dangerous because infections could
be treated successfully. The discovery of penicillin also led to the development of many new classes and compounds of antibiotics. However, as discussed in Chapter 11, some of the medical gains achieved by the introduction
of penicillin are now considered to be under threat because many types of
bacteria have developed resistance to antibiotics.

Disease eradication campaigns

Health services and programmes delivered through a country's existing
health system, which seeks to address the population's overall health needs
on a long-term basis, are sometimes known as horizontal or integrated health
programmes. These include health promotion and vaccination services provided through community-based services and primary care facilities, as well
as secondary care services, such as specialist outpatient care and hospitals.
Another approach that has frequently been used to control communicable
disease is that of targeted, disease-specific campaigns. These are often
known as vertical health programmes. However, it is misleading to suggest
there is a dichotomy between vertical and horizontal approaches. In practice,
communicable disease control often involves a combination of the two
approaches, with some activities well integrated into mainstream health services and others delivered as part of separate disease-specific interventions.
In each context, the combination of approaches depends on local health
system structures and capacities and the problems that are being addressed
(Atun et al., 2009).

Some disease-specific campaigns have attempted to eradicate specific
communicable diseases. Eradication is defined as the permanent reduction to zero of the worldwide incidence of infection. One such example is
the campaign to eradicate smallpox. Smallpox is an acute contagious
disease caused by the variola virus, a member of the orthopoxvirus family.
For the virus to be sustained in a population, it must pass from person to

person in a continuing chain of infection, and is spread by inhalation of air droplets or aerosols (Henderson, 1999). Smallpox is one of the most devastating infectious diseases ever. It has a mortality rate of around 30% and between 65% and 80% of survivors are marked with deep-pitted scars. Although an effective vaccine had existed for over a century, a lack of global coordination to ensure systematic control of outbreaks and vaccination meant that in the 1950s there continued to be an estimated 50 million cases of smallpox every year. The World Health Assembly, the governing body of the WHO, voted to support a global smallpox eradication campaign in 1959. The original idea was for individual countries to take the lead with technical support from WHO. However, despite these early efforts, smallpox was still circulating in 31 countries in 1966.

The Intensified Smallpox Eradication Campaign was launched in 1966, under the leadership of the WHO. The campaign involved a globally coordinated strategy involving mass vaccination, surveillance and containment measures. Figure 1.3 shows a poster illustrating the many different activities of the Smallpox Eradication Programme in Ethiopia in the 1970s. It was clear that as long as any cases of disease remained, it could reappear anywhere. This was demonstrated in 1972 in an outbreak in Kosovo, then

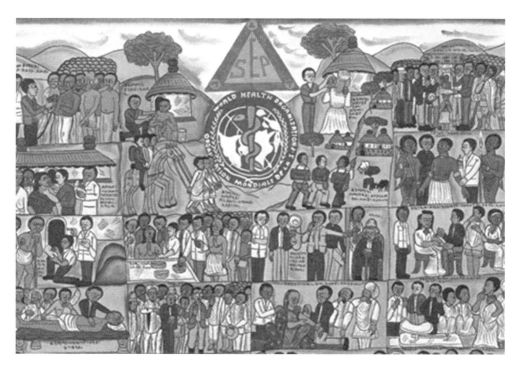

Figure 1.3 Ethiopian poster illustrating the activities of the Smallpox Eradication Programme, 1970s
Source: WHO.

part of the Socialist Federal Republic of Yugoslavia in Eastern Europe, which infected 175 people and killed 35. At that time Europe was thought to be free of smallpox. The response was a drive to vaccinate the whole population, a total of 21 million people. The teams worked so fast that 18 million were vaccinated in just 10 days (WHO, 2011). The last case of naturally occurring smallpox was in Somalia in 1977. As a result of the success of the Intensified Smallpox Eradication Campaign, smallpox was declared eradicated in 1980. Smallpox is regarded as the most successful eradication campaign against a communicable disease.

Other eradication campaigns have targeted diseases such as malaria and polio. However, so far these have proved more challenging for a number of reasons. The WHO began the Global Malaria Eradication Program (GMEP) in 1955. During the GMEP, malaria was permanently eliminated from many regions. However, in the 1960s, not only did some areas fail to advance as expected, but other areas saw resurgences of malaria after relatively long periods of interruption of transmission. In 1969, the WHO recognized that there were countries where eradication was not feasible in the short term, and that a strategy of disease control was an appropriate step towards future eradication in those areas. Reasons for the failure of the eradication campaign include an oversimplified strategy that did not take sufficient account of local contexts, the emergence of resistance to insecticides, lack of health system capacity for case detection and management in some areas, and insufficient community engagement in others (Nájera et al., 2011). More recently, the WHO shifted the focus of efforts from eradication to preventing the re-establishment of malaria in all countries that are malaria-free, reducing malaria mortality, reducing malaria case incidence and eliminating malaria in at least 35 countries, with elimination defined as the interruption of local transmission of a specified malaria parasite in a defined geographic area (WHO, 2016c).

The Global Polio Eradication Initiative was formed in 1988. At that time, polio paralysed more than 350,000 people a year. The programme was initially very successful and the disease disappeared from many countries. However, tackling the last 1% of polio cases proved to be difficult. Conflicts, political instability, hard-to-reach populations and poor infrastructure presented huge challenges, with different circumstances in each country requiring local solutions. In 2013, the Global Polio Eradication Initiative launched a comprehensive strategic plan that outlined measures for eliminating polio in its last strongholds and for maintaining a polio-free world. By 2015, all countries but two had stopped polio transmission, and in that year there were just 74 cases of polio. However, without full eradication, cases of polio could quickly increase and the disease could reappear in countries that are currently polio-free. The Global Polio Eradication Initiative developed an Endgame Strategic Plan, which outlines how it intends to complete the eradication of the disease and certify the eradication (Global Polio Eradication Initiative, 2013).

While some disease eradication campaigns have not proven successful, the initiatives have reduced the burden of disease. They have marked a trend towards international collaboration and support, reflecting an understanding of the need to coordinate such campaigns globally with strong leadership and adequate funding. In addition, these campaigns have provided valuable lessons about community engagement, cultural sensitivity and the importance of working with existing health and social systems that have been used by other communicable disease control programmes.

✎ Activity 1.1

Read the following extract taken from *Bugs, drugs and smoke: Stories from public health* (WHO, 2011), then consider the questions that follow.

Dr Halfdan Mahler, WHO director-general at the time, later described the smallpox programme as 'a triumph of management, not of medicine'. But given the numerous problems that had to be overcome, including shortages of funds and vaccine, dysfunctional or non-existent national health services, infected refugees fleeing civil war and famine, traditional beliefs, and all the problems posed by climate and difficult terrain, it might be said that the programme was also an extraordinary triumph of the human will.

1. What factors do you think contributed to the success of the Intensified Smallpox Eradication Campaign?
2. Are there any specific features of smallpox that you think made it feasible for it to be eradicated? If so, what are those features?

Feedback

1. Factors that contributed to the success of the Intensified Smallpox Eradication Campaign include: a strategy that involved mass vaccination as well as surveillance and control; centralized funding; global leadership from the WHO; increased understanding of community beliefs; acknowledgement of local context factors and adaptation to these; availability of resources to respond immediately to outbreaks; and availability of effective vaccines.
2. Features of an infectious disease that might potentially allow it to be eradicated include: there is an effective intervention to interrupt transmission, such as a vaccine; there are practical diagnostic tools to detect the disease; and humans are essential for the survival of the microorganism causing the disease, so it cannot persist and multiply in other animals or in the environment. You might also have said

that as new tools are developed, it may become feasible for other diseases to be eradicated. You may also have referred to practical considerations such as availability of funding, leadership, human resources, broad social and community support for eradication, a feasible and acceptable strategy, the impact of the disease warrants the investment of eradication (in terms of cost-effectiveness and social benefits), and political support at national and international levels (Miller *et al.*, 2006).

The emergence of HIV and public health activism

In June 1981, the Centers for Disease Control and Prevention (CDC) in the USA reported in its Morbidity and Mortality Weekly Report unusual clusters of a rare lung infection called pneumocystis carinii pneumonia (PCP) in previously healthy young men. Those affected also had other unusual infections, indicating that their immune systems were not working properly. This marked the first official reporting of what became known as the acquired immune deficiency syndrome (AIDS) epidemic. Some researchers began calling the condition 'gay-related immune deficiency' (GRID) because many of the individuals affected were men who have sex with men (MSM). In 1982, CDC first used the term AIDS because scientists recognized that the disease was not restricted to gay men. In 1983, researchers at the Pasteur Institute in Paris reported that they had isolated a new retrovirus, a type of virus, that they believed caused AIDS. Further research in the USA confirmed this and in 1986 the retrovirus was named Human Immunodeficiency Virus (HIV).

Many people living with HIV may experience stigma and discrimination. Stigma, in this context, is defined as negative beliefs, feelings and attitudes towards people living with HIV, groups associated with people living with HIV and other key populations at higher risk of HIV infection. Discrimination refers to the unfair and unjust treatment of an individual based on his or her real or perceived HIV status (UNAIDS, 2014). Research has shown that this stigma and discrimination undermines HIV prevention efforts by making people afraid to seek HIV information and services to reduce their risk of infection (UNAIDS, 2014). In the early years after its identification, HIV was often referred to as 'the gay plague' as it was believed to mean certain death and so caused extreme fear. In addition, people with HIV were often blamed for their infection because it was associated with actions that some people disapprove of, such as drug use and particular sexual behaviours. People with HIV throughout the world have had difficulty accessing care, support and basic services. For example, there are press reports of funeral care providers refusing to provide services for people who died as a result of AIDS in the USA (Bass, 1987).

In the early 1980s, a movement of activists campaigning for funding and research into treatment for HIV emerged in the USA. These activists challenged the stigma and discrimination experienced by people living with HIV and demanded to be treated as equal partners in ongoing research. New organizations were set up, such as Act-Up (The AIDS Coalition to Unleash Power) and TAG (Treatment Action Group), which demanded government agencies, pharmaceutical companies and the medical establishment prioritize research into treatment and provide services for people living with HIV (France, 2016). These organizations used direct action, media campaigns and other forms of advocacy and provided information, advice and support services to people living with HIV. In some cases, this included providing access to HIV treatment through 'buyers clubs', which enabled people to purchase medications themselves before it was licensed by government authorities. This activist movement spread worldwide and exists today in the form of thousands of national and local non-governmental organizations NGOs advocating on behalf of people living with HIV. It is credited with making a crucial contribution to speeding up the development of effective treatments for HIV and making these available to millions of people globally (UNAIDS, 2011).

However, despite advances in treatment that have significantly reduced AIDS-related mortality in recent years, the pandemic is far from over. Many people living with HIV still do not have access to treatment. In addition, in 2015 there were 2.1 million new HIV infections worldwide, giving a total of 36.7 million people living with HIV (UNAIDS, 2016).

✎ Activity 1.2

In 1962, Sir McFarland Burnett, an eminent virologist, stated: 'By the end of the Second World War it was possible to say that almost all of the major practical problems of dealing with infectious disease had been solved' (Brachman, 2003).

- What practical problems do you think he is referring to? Were these solved and, if so, how?
- Do you agree with the statement? If not, why do you think infectious disease is still a health issue?

Feedback

The practical problems you could have included in your response are: not accurately understanding what causes infectious diseases; lack of effective treatment; inability to prevent infection; inability to identify the source of infection; inadequate sanitation; fear and stigma of disease.

Solutions you could have included in your response are: germ theory; epidemiology; immunization; sanitation and hygiene improvements; public health; antibiotics; new environmental controls such as insecticides.

Reasons you may have included in your response as to why infectious disease is still a health issue include: the emergence of new infections such as HIV; growing resistance to antibiotics and insecticides; poor public health and healthcare infrastructure in many parts of the world, so control of communicable disease is inadequate; high levels of poverty and poor baseline health, so people are susceptible to infection; conflicts and natural disasters that disrupt usual communicable disease control; poor living conditions in many parts of the world, so infections thrive and spread quickly; and changing social, economic and ecological factors such as increased population mobility/air travel, land-use change, climate change and agricultural intensification, which can drive the emergence and spread of infectious diseases.

Changes in health outcomes

Health outcomes, including life expectancy, improved significantly in the nineteenth and twentieth centuries. Improvements in life expectancy have been greater and began to happen earlier in countries that industrialized first, especially in Western Europe and North America. Life expectancy in other regions started to increase more rapidly in the 1950s, as shown in Table 1.1.

Over the period of 1841 to 2009 data for England and Wales show, male and female life expectancy at birth increased from 40.6 to 78.4 years and from 42.3 to 82.5 years respectively, with significant short-term decreases during the First World War, the influenza pandemic of 1918/19 and the Second World War (Longevity Science Advisory Panel, 2012). In the nineteenth century, poor life expectancy at birth was largely due to the very high rates of infant and childhood mortality. In the 1840s, around 15% of babies died before their first birthday compared with 0.4% in 2009. Survival past the first year of life was historically a predominant factor in life expectancies and once a child had reached five years of age, he or she was much more likely to reach a greater age. Historically, infectious diseases were the major causes of childhood morbidity and mortality. The developments in communicable disease control outlined in this chapter made a significant contribution to reducing infant and childhood mortality and, in doing so, increasing life expectancy at birth.

During the nineteenth and twentieth centuries, there were also changes in the main causes of mortality and morbidity. Table 1.2 shows the top ten causes of death in the USA in 1900 and 2010. Infectious diseases now

Table 1.1 Life expectancy at birth (males and females combined): trends from 1950 to 2015, by United Nations (UN) region and World

UN region	1950–55	1955–60	1960–65	1965–70	1970–75	1975–80	1980–85	1985–90	1990–95	1995–2000	2000–05	2005–10	2010–15
Africa	37.34	39.85	42.22	44.31	46.40	48.60	50.50	51.77	51.73	52.25	53.29	56.49	59.55
Asia	42.10	44.34	46.30	52.63	56.37	59.19	61.42	63.45	65.08	66.57	68.51	70.14	71.57
Europe	63.59	67.07	69.17	70.02	70.60	71.02	71.63	72.81	72.60	73.06	73.76	75.26	77.01
Latin America	51.22	54.14	56.78	58.95	61.16	63.00	64.85	66.63	68.40	70.45	72.15	73.40	74.54
North America	68.59	69.67	70.15	70.45	71.38	73.24	74.43	75.00	75.82	76.60	77.37	78.36	79.16
Oceania	60.45	62.45	63.86	65.05	66.38	68.19	70.17	70.90	72.51	73.63	75.14	76.64	77.47
World	46.81	49.21	51.07	55.38	58.05	60.21	62.00	63.61	64.54	65.58	67.04	68.85	70.47

Source: United Nations, Department of Economic and Social Affairs, Population Division (2015).

Table 1.2 Top 10 causes of death in the USA (no. of deaths per 100,000)

	1900	2010
1	Pneumonia or influenza (202.2)	Heart disease (192.9)
2	Tuberculosis (194.4)	Cancer (185.9)
3	Gastrointestinal infections (142.7)	Non-infectious airways diseases (44.6)
4	Heart disease (137.4)	Cerebrovascular disease (41.8)
5	Cerebrovascular disease (106.9)	Accidents (38.2)
6	Nephropathies (88.6)	Alzheimer's disease (27)
7	Accidents (72.3)	Diabetes (22.3)
8	Cancer (64)	Nephropathies (16.3)
9	Senility (50.2)	Pneumonia or influenza (16.2)
10	Diphtheria (40.3)	Suicide (12.2)

Source: Data are from the Centers for Disease Control and Prevention (CDC).

account for many fewer deaths than in the nineteenth and early twentieth centuries. Non-communicable diseases, sometimes known as chronic diseases, have come to represent a much more significant cause of mortality. These non-communicable diseases usually affect older people and are associated with social, economic, environmental and lifestyle factors, including poor air quality, poverty, bad housing, poor diet, lack of exercise and tobacco use. Importantly, they cause very significant morbidity as well as mortality. The burden of disease has shifted from premature death, and particularly infant mortality, from infectious diseases, to people living longer with chronic conditions. This shift has been referred to as the epidemiological transition (Omran, 1971).

Collectively, the developments in communicable disease control outlined above played a part in creating the conditions for this epidemiological transition. It is not possible to assign relative importance to one development over another. Rather, in many cases, one development enabled another and they interacted to generate improvements in outcomes. Other factors also contributed. For example, improved standards of living, and especially diet, are likely to have contributed to a decline in TB rates before the introduction of antibiotics (Jones *et al*., 2012). It is also important to acknowledge that the pace of progress has not been universal. Communicable diseases continue to cause substantial mortality and morbidity in low-income countries, where respiratory infections, HIV/AIDS, diarrheal diseases, malaria and TB combined account for almost one-third of all deaths (WHO, 2017).

Summary

There is evidence that many of the infectious diseases of modern human populations also affected ancient civilizations. Other infectious diseases have emerged more recently. While reliable figures on mortality from infectious diseases do not exist for older civilizations, population growth, denser living conditions and increased movement of people are likely to have made them more numerous, widespread and deadly. Some of the mechanisms of communicable disease control in use today have their origins in the ancient or medieval periods. However, most were developed in the nineteenth and twentieth centuries, including germ theory, public health, epidemiology, immunization, vertical disease control and eradication programmes. More recently, the emergence of HIV and the growth of activism have had a profound impact on communicable disease control. These developments in communicable disease control have contributed to substantial improvements in health outcomes. However, challenges remain and new threats are emerging. These will be discussed in the final chapter of this book.

Further reading

Berridge, V., Gorsky, M. and Mold, A. (2011) *Public Health in History*. Maidenhead: Open University Press.

References

Acheson, D. (1988) *Public Health in England: The Report of the Committee of Inquiry into the Future Development of the Public Health Function*. London: HMSO.

Amulree, Lord (1973) Hygienic conditions in ancient Rome and modern London, *Medical History (Great Britain)*, 17 (3): 244–255.

Angelakis, A., Kavoulaki, E. and Dialynas, E. (2014) Sanitation and wastewater technologies in Minoan Era, in A.N. Angelakis and J.B. Rose (eds.) *Evolution of Sanitation and Wastewater Technologies through the Centuries* (pp. 1–24). London: IWA Publishing.

Atun, R., de Jongh, T., Secci, F.V., Ohiri, K. and Adeyi, O. (2009) *Clearing the global health fog: A systematic review of the evidence on integration of health systems and targeted intervention*, Working Paper #166. Washington, DC: The World Bank.

Bass, S. (1987) Funeral homes accused of bias on aids, *New York Times*, 15 November. Available at: http://www.nytimes.com/1987/11/15/nyregion/funeral-homes-accused-of-bias-on-aids.html

Blevins, S.M. and Bronze, M.S. (2010) Robert Koch and the 'golden age' of bacteriology, *International Journal of Infectious Diseases*, 14 (9): e744–e751.

Brachman, P.S. (2003) Infectious diseases – past, present, and future, *International Journal of Epidemiology*, 32 (5): 684–686.

Cameron, D. and Jones, I.G. (1983) John Snow, the Broad Street pump and modern epidemiology, *International Journal of Epidemiology*, 12 (4): 393–396.

Deng, Y. (2011) *Ancient Chinese Inventions*. Cambridge: Cambridge University Press.

Dinc, G. and Ulman, Y.I. (2007). The introduction of variolation 'A La Turca' to the West by Lady Mary Montagu and Turkey's contribution to this, *Vaccine*, 25 (21): 4261–4265.

Donajgrodzki, A.P. (ed.) (1977) *Social Control in Nineteenth Century Britain*. London: Croom Helm.

Dowdle, W.R. and Cochi, S.L. (2011) The principles and feasibility of disease eradication, *Vaccine*, 29 (suppl. 4): D70–D73.

France, D. (2016) *How to Survive a Plague: The Inside Story of How Citizens and Science Tamed AIDS*. New York: Knopf.

Global Polio Eradication Initiative (2013) *Polio eradication and endgame strategic plan 2013–2018*, Fact File. Available at: http://polioeradication.org/wp-content/uploads/2016/07/GPEI_Plan_FactFile_EN-1.pdf.

Gottfried, R.S. (2010) *The Black Death*. New York: Simon & Schuster.

Greenwood, D. (2007) *Antimicrobial Chemotherapy*. New York: Oxford University Press.

Hamlin, C. (1998) *Public Health and Social Justice in the Age of Chadwick, Britain 1800–1854*. Cambridge: Cambridge University Press.

Henderson, D.A. (1999) Smallpox: clinical and epidemiologic features, *Emerging Infectious Diseases*, 5 (4): 537–539.

Hershkovitz, I., Donoghue, H.D., Minnikin, D.E., Besra, G.S., Lee, O.Y.-C., Gernaey, A.M. *et al.* (2008) Detection and molecular characterization of 9,000-year-old *Mycobacterium tuberculosis* from a Neolithic settlement in the Eastern Mediterranean, *PLoS One*, 3 (10): e3426.

Jones, D.S., Podolsky, S.H. and Greene, J.A. (2012) The burden of disease and the changing task of medicine, *New England Journal of Medicine*, 366 (25): 2333–2338.

Jones, S. (2016) *Germs, genes and genesis: The history of infectious disease*, Gresham College Lecture at the Museum of London, 16 February 2016. Transcript available at: https://www.gresham.ac.uk/lectures-and-events/germs-genes-and-genesis-the-history-of-infectious-disease#pJYSl3jmHTYb8OQh.99.

Lederberg, J. (2000) Infectious history, *Science*, 288 (5464): 287–293.

Ligon, B.L. (2004) Penicillin: its discovery and early development, *Seminars in Pediatric Infectious Diseases*, 15 (1): 52–57.

Longevity Science Advisory Panel (2012) *Life expectancy: Past and future variations by gender in England and Wales*, LSAP Paper #2. Available at: http://www.longevitypanel.co.uk/_files/life-expectancy-by-gender.pdf

Mackowiak, P.A. and Sehdev, P.S. (2002) The origin of quarantine, *Clinical Infectious Diseases*, 35 (9): 1071–1072.

Merriam-Webster (2016) *Merriam-Webster's Medical Dictionary*, New Edition. Springfield, MA: Merriam-Webster, Inc.

Miller, M., Barrett, S. and Henderson, D.A. (2006) Control and eradication, in D.T. Jamison, J.G. Breman, A.R. Measham, G. Alleyne, M. Claeson, D.B. Evans *et al.* (eds.) *Disease Control Priorities in Developing Countries*, 2nd edn. Washington, DC: The International Bank for Reconstruction and Development/The World Bank and New York: Oxford University Press. Available at: https://www.ncbi.nlm.nih.gov/books/NBK11763/.

Nájera, J.A., González-Silva, M. and Alonso, P.L. (2011) Some lessons for the future from the Global Malaria Eradication Programme (1955–1969), *PLoS Medicine*, 8 (1): e1000412.

Nwaozuzu, E.E. and Ebi, G.C. (2014) Antimicrobial screening and therapeutic potentials of crude extracts of plants used as anti-malarial remedies in Ibo-Nigeria folkloric medicine, *Journal of Biology, Agriculture and Healthcare*, 4 (25): 27–31.

Omran, A.R. (1971) The epidemiologic transition: a theory of the epidemiology of population change, *The Milbank Memorial Fund Quarterly*, 49 (4): 509–38. Reprinted 2005 in *The Milbank Quarterly*, 83 (4): 731–757.

Quinn, R. (2013) Rethinking antibiotic research and development: World War II and the Penicillin Collaborative, *American Journal of Public Health*, 103 (3): 426–434.

Riedel, S. (2005) Edward Jenner and the history of smallpox and vaccination, *Proceedings (Baylor University. Medical Center)*, 18 (1): 21–25.

Robbins, G., Tripathy, V.M., Misra, V.N., Mohanty, R.K., Shinde, V.S., Gray, K.M. *et al.* (2009) Ancient skeletal evidence for leprosy in India (2000 B.C.), *PLoS One*, 4 (5): e5669.

Ryle, J.A. (1948) *Changing Disciplines*. London: Oxford University Press.

Tognotti, E. (2013) Lessons from the history of quarantine, from plague to influenza A, *Emerging Infectious Diseases*, 19 (2): 254–259.

UNAIDS (2011) *UNAIDS guidance for partnerships with civil society, including people living with HIV and key populations*, UNAIDS Guidance Document. Geneva: UNAIDS. Available at: http://www.unaids. org/sites/default/files/media_asset/JC2236_guidance_partnership_civilsociety_en_0.pdf.

UNAIDS (2014) *Reduction of HIV-related stigma and discrimination*, UNAIDS Guidance Note. Geneva: UNAIDS. Available at: http://www.unaids.org/sites/default/files/media_asset/2014unaidsguidancenote_ stigma_en.pdf.

UNAIDS (2016) *Global AIDS update 2016*. Geneva: UNAIDS. Available at: http://www.unaids.org/sites/ default/files/media_asset/global-AIDS-update-2016_en.pdf.

United Nations, Department of Economic and Social Affairs, Population Division (2015) *World population prospects: The 2015 revision*, custom data acquired via website.

Wolfe, N.D., Dunavan, C.P. and Diamond, J. (2007) Origins of major human infectious diseases, *Nature*, 447 (7142): 279–283.

World Health Organization (WHO) (2011) *Bugs, drugs and smoke: Stories from public health*. Geneva: WHO. Available at: http://www.who.int/about/history/publications/public_health_stories/en/.

World Health Organization (WHO) (2013) *Global vaccine action plan 2011–2020*. Geneva: WHO. Available at: http://www.who.int/immunization/global_vaccine_action_plan/GVAP_doc_2011_2020/en/.

World Health Organization (WHO) (2016a) *Tetanus*, Fact Sheet. Geneva: WHO. Available at: http://www. who.int/immunization/diseases/tetanus/en/ [accessed 30 January 2017].

World Health Organization (WHO) (2016b) *Health topic: Hygiene*. Geneva: WHO. Available at: http:// www.who.int/topics/hygiene/en/.

World Health Organization (WHO) (2016c) *Eliminating malaria*. Geneva: WHO. Available at: http://www. who.int/malaria/publications/atoz/eliminating-malaria/en/.

World Health Organization (WHO) (2017) *The top 10 causes of death*, Fact Sheet. Available at: http:// www.who.int/mediacentre/factsheets/fs310/en/index2.html.

2

Concepts in communicable disease causation

Liza Cragg

Overview

In order to develop and to apply effective control measures for communicable disease, it is essential to understand the factors that contribute to the cause of such diseases. This chapter introduces the epidemiological triad, a model that conceptualizes communicable disease causation as an interaction of factors relating to agent, host and environment. It then describes the different types of agents that can cause infectious disease and the factors that influence whether a person develops a disease, including how marginalization can increase vulnerability to communicable disease. The chapter also explains the terminology frequently used in communicable disease control and how these terms are applied in this book.

Learning objectives

After reading this chapter, you will be able to:

- explain the epidemiological triad and how it is used to conceptualize the causes of communicable disease
- identify the major types of infectious agents, and describe the key features of each type
- identify the factors that influence whether individuals are susceptible to disease
- explain how marginalization can increase vulnerability to communicable disease

Key terms

Host: A person, animal or other organism that becomes infected by a pathogen.

Infection: The entry and development of an infectious agent in the body of a person or animal, which may be either apparent (causing symptoms) or inapparent (causing no symptoms).

Infectivity: The ability of an agent to enter and replicate in a host.

Marginalized community: A group that is on the fringes of a society or population because of a lack of rights, resources and opportunities.

Pathogenicity: The ability of an agent to cause disease in a host.

Reservoir: Any person, animal or plant (or any population or community of one or more species of these organisms), or any soil or substance, where an infectious agent can survive and multiply, and from where it can be transmitted to a susceptible host.

Transmission: Any mechanism through which an infectious agent is spread between hosts or from a reservoir to a host.

Vector: Any living organism which transfers an infectious agent from one host to another.

Virulence: The extent of disease an agent can cause in a host.

Zoonoses or zoonotic diseases: Infections that are naturally transmissible from vertebrate animals to humans and vice versa.

Communicable disease causation

The most commonly used model for conceptualizing the causes of infectious diseases is the epidemiological triad. This model consists of an agent, a host and an environment. The agent is a substance or organism that is capable of producing infection. Infectious agents are sometimes referred to as pathogens. The host refers to the organism, which could be human, animal or plant, that can contract the disease, depending on its exposure and susceptibility. The environment is made up of external factors that affect the host and the agent. Disease results when the environment enables the agent to interact with a susceptible host. The ability of an agent to enter and replicate in a host is known as its infectivity. The ability of an agent to cause disease is referred to as its pathogenicity. The extent of disease caused by an agent in a host is referred to as virulence, with highly virulent diseases able to cause extremely serious and deadly diseases. Virulence is affected by host and environment. Two ways of illustrating the epidemiological triad, as a triangle and as a Venn diagram, are shown in Figure 2.1.

The control of communicable disease involves public policy interventions that restrict the circulation of an infectious agent beyond the level that would result from spontaneous, individual behaviours to protect against infection (Barrett, 2004). As this book goes on to explain, mechanisms to control communicable disease include interventions that address the environment, the host and the infectious agent.

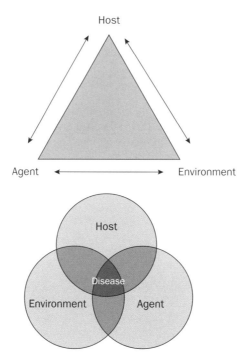

Figure 2.1 The epidemiologic triad, shown as a triangle and as a Venn diagram

---

✎ **Activity 2.1**

Make a list of the different communicable diseases that you have been affected by. What do you think caused them? When you have finished reading this chapter, return to your list. What can you add now to your explanation of what might have caused these diseases?

Feedback

You might have included common communicable diseases that most people contract such as the common cold (rhinovirus), flu (influenza virus) or food- or water-borne infections. You might also have contracted, or know someone in your family or community who has contracted, a vaccine-preventable disease such as measles or rubella. Depending on where you live, some mosquito-borne diseases, such as malaria and dengue fever, may be endemic in your country.

Infectious agents

Infectious agents that cause disease fall into the following main groups: bacteria, viruses, protozoa, helminths and fungi (Janeway *et al.*, 2001). Recent research has identified prions as an additional type of infectious agent. The key features of each group of infectious agents are described in more detail below.

Bacteria

Bacteria are microorganisms that can cause infectious disease. Bacteria typically live in colonies. Bacterium is the singular of bacteria. While bacteria sometimes cause diseases, they are also responsible for a variety of essential functions in the body, including digestion and the extraction of energy from nutrients. Recent research suggests that there are a similar number of bacteria in the human body as there are human cells (Sender *et al.*, 2016). Many bacteria live on other organisms to the mutual benefit of both the host organism and the bacterium, which is known as mutualism. In some cases, the bacteria benefit but cause neither harm nor benefit to the host organism, which is known as commensalism. However, if the host organism's innate immune defences are disturbed, previously harmless bacteria can become harmful.

Taxonomy of bacteria

Taxonomy is the science of defining groups of biological organisms on the basis of shared characteristics and giving names to those groups. Bacteria are classified using the same method of defining groups with shared characteristics as used for all life on Earth. These groups are:

1. Domain
2. Kingdom
3. Phylum
4. Class
5. Order
6. Family
7. Genus
8. Species

As the taxonomy descends from 1 to 8, the groups become more similar and smaller. In bacterial taxonomy, a number of functional considerations determine the name applied to a bacterial species. These include: its shape; how it is identified in the laboratory (for example, gram staining); where it can live and thrive (for example, its oxygen requirements); and common reservoirs (that is, where specific bacteria are likely to reside). Naming bacterial species is crucial, as it enables understanding of features of particular bacteria to be shared across disciplines. In bacteriology, the names used for bacterial species are very descriptive, so they are able to convey a lot of information concisely. Case study 2.1 describes Streptococci, which are Gram-positive bacteria that cause many common infectious diseases in humans, in more detail.

Shape of bacteria

The names of bacterial species are often related strongly to the shape of the organisms, as illustrated in Figure 2.2. There are three basic shapes of bacteria; cocci, which are round; bacilli, which are rod shaped; and spirillum, which are spiral shaped or can appear coiled. Although bacteria often exist as solitary cells, some types join together in pairs, chains or grape-like clusters.

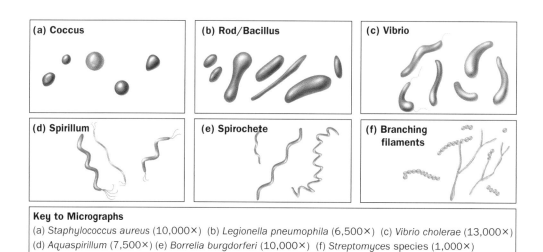

Key to Micrographs
(a) *Staphylococcus aureus* (10,000×) (b) *Legionella pneumophila* (6,500×) (c) *Vibrio cholerae* (13,000×)
(d) *Aquaspirillum* (7,500×) (e) *Borrelia burgdorferi* (10,000×) (f) *Streptomyces* species (1,000×)

Figure 2.2 Shapes of bacteria
Source: Talaro and Chess (2017).

Gram staining of bacteria

Microbiologists often refer to bacteria as being Gram-negative or Gram-positive. This refers to how an organism reacts to a dye, or stain, used to identify bacteria in the laboratory. It is named after the bacteriologist Hans Christian Gram who developed the technique. The Gram stain is often the first stage undertaken to identify bacteria. The dye, which is crystal violet, is added to the sample and then diluted with various agents. Gram-positive organisms retain the violet in their cell walls, which indicates the presence of a thick layer of peptidoglycan, a polymer of amino acids and sugars that makes up the cell wall of all bacteria. Gram-negative cells stain red, which indicates a thin layer of peptidoglycan leading to less retention of the violet dye. Although many types of bacteria are grouped as being Gram-positive or Gram-negative, not all bacteria respond predictably to Gram staining, so some cannot be classified into either of these groups and are referred to as Gram-indeterminate bacteria.

Oxygen requirements of bacteria

Bacteria that live and grow in oxygen-rich environments are known as aerobic bacteria. These bacteria use aerobic respiration and break down glucose to release energy. Bacteria that live and grow in environments where oxygen is absent are known as anaerobic bacteria. These bacteria survive by producing their energy requirements through anaerobic fermentation. However, these criteria are not dichotomous, as some bacteria are capable of switching between aerobic respiration and anaerobic fermentation, depending on whether oxygen is present in their environment. These bacteria are known as facultative anaerobes. Understanding the oxygen requirements of bacteria causing an infection is important in determining how to treat it. In general, anaerobic bacteria are more challenging to treat.

Bacterial reservoirs

A reservoir is a place where microorganisms exist naturally and multiply. It can be a person, an animal, a plant (or a group, population or community of individuals from one or more species of these organisms), or soil or another substance. When the reservoir is a living organism, the bacteria's presence is often as a commensal organism; the host organism is not normally harmed by the presence of the bacteria. A reservoir can also be an individual who is infected by bacteria. When bacteria are living on or in a host organism without causing harm, the organism is said to be colonized by that bacteria. Importantly, being colonized by bacteria is not the same as being infected by bacteria. Infection denotes that bacteria have invaded tissue and are causing damage, whereas colonization means that the bacteria are present but not having a negative impact on the body.

Case study 2.1:   Streptococci

Streptococci are Gram-positive bacteria, which resemble balls bound together in long chain sequences. Streptococci are classified as alpha-haemolytic, beta-haemolytic or non-haemolytic, which refers to their presentation on the blood agar plate used to grow them. Alpha-haemolytic streptococci include *Streptococcus pneumoniae*, which is responsible for pneumonia and many other infections. Beta-haemolytic streptococci are classified in groups A to H. They include *Streptococcus pyogenes*, which is the leading cause of 'strep throat', and *Streptococcus bovis*, which can cause an infection of the lining of the heart. Both groups A and B beta-haemolytic streptococci are common commensal organisms found in humans. Group A beta-haemolytic streptococci are found often in the nose, throat, vagina and rectum. Group B beta-haemolytic streptococci can be found in the vagina, cervix, urethra, skin and throat. Colonization with these organisms is normal, and is not a cause for concern. However, there is a risk of infection when these bacteria are able to evade the body's innate immune defences, as when a person's immune system is suppressed.

Viruses

Viruses are another type of infectious agent. There are important differences between bacteria and viruses. Viruses are much smaller than bacteria. A virus does not have its own cellular structure; instead, it replicates inside the cells of other living organisms. Viruses can infect all life forms, including animals, plants and microorganisms. Our understanding of the origins of viruses, their functions and their characteristics is still developing. Recent research has revealed the global spread of an ancient group of retroviruses that affected about 28 of 50 modern mammals' ancestors some 15–30 million years ago (Diehl *et al.*, 2016). In addition, research is identifying opportunities to use viruses in genetic engineering and for the treatment of certain diseases (Sze *et al.*, 2013). Bacteria and viruses also behave differently. Whereas bacterial infections tend to infect and cause disease in a single organ or body part, viruses usually affect a number of organs or the entire body in what is known as systemic infection.

Classification of viruses

Viruses are classified using the Baltimore Classification depending on the type of genome. There are three major types: DNA, RNA and reverse tran scribing viruses. These types are further divided into seven groups, according to the number of DNA or RNA strands present, and the polarity (positive or negative) of the strand, or 'sense'. Groups I and II are DNA viruses, groups III–V are RNA viruses, while groups VI–VII are reverse transcribing viruses. Examples of diseases caused by DNA viruses are varicella (chickenpox) and herpes. Rubella and Ebola viral disease are caused by RNA viruses. HIV and hepatitis B are caused by reverse transcribing viruses.

Identification of viruses

Unlike bacteria, viruses cannot be seen with a light microscope. The identification of viruses is far more complex and, depending on the technique used, costly. Given that viruses are not able to survive and replicate outside of a host cell, they must be cultured in living tissues. The major techniques used to isolate, grow and identify viruses are as follows.

- *Culturing bacteriophages*: Bacteriophages are viruses that infect and multiply within bacteria. The bacteria eventually die and the pattern of cell death enables identification by microbiologists.
- *Animal inoculation*: Laboratory animals can be inoculated with virus samples, which allow viruses to infect the animals and grow. Researchers then observe the animals for signs of disease, and isolate the multiplied virus from tissues. There are risks and limitations associated with this method, including the potential for mutation and viral escape; differences in how human viruses behave in laboratory animals; and the ethics of using live animals for experimentation.
- *Embryo inoculation*: Embryo inoculation involves injecting the embryos of certain animals with live viruses. The viruses are able to infect and multiply in the tissues of these embryonic cells for later identification.
- *Cell culture*: Cell culture is a complex but very efficient way of growing viruses and conducting vaccine research. The process involves growing specific types of animal cells in culture media. The cells are infected with viruses, which cause observable changes in the cultures.
- *Clinical testing*: Additional clinical tests exist for the identification of certain viruses. These tests include rapid test kits, which detect the presence of certain viruses or antibodies to them. Common examples include test kits for influenza and human immunodeficiency virus (HIV). Molecular tests, such as polymerase chain reaction (PCR), are commonly used in clinical settings to test for specific viral material. PCR testing requires costly equipment and trained laboratory technicians, making it challenging to use in resource-limited settings.

Viral reservoirs

The most common reservoirs for viruses are humans or animals. Some viruses have the potential to cross over between animals and humans to cause disease – these are known as zoonotic viral diseases. Some of the diseases that have emerged recently, such as HIV and Ebola virus diseases (EVD), are zoonotic viral diseases.

Protozoa

Protozoa are a diverse group of single-celled organisms. Most protozoa have mechanisms to support movement, such as a flagella or cilia, and require external nutrients, as they are not capable of synthesizing their own food. Protozoa play an important ecological role, as they consume bacteria for food and act as an important source of nutrients for higher-level microscopic organisms. Malaria is an example of an infectious disease caused by protozoan parasites, which infect humans using mosquitoes as the vector. Not all protozoan organisms require vectors of transmission. Cryptosporidium is a protozoan parasite, spread typically through faecal–oral transmission, often via a contaminated water supply. There are a wide variety of protozoan species and they can be found in many different reservoirs. Given the diversity of protozoa, it is essential to understand the reservoir and mechanism of transmission of the particular infectious agent. This allows for preventative action, such as vector control or water sanitation, to stop people from becoming infected or spreading the parasite further.

Protozoa shapes

Protozoa are broadly classified according to their shape:

- *Amoebae*: Amoebae, like all protozoa, are single-celled organisms. Unlike other protozoa, amoebae do not have any one fixed shape. They are shape shifters, able to alter their shape as required.
- *Flagellates*: Flagellates are identified by the presence of a tail-like structure or structures, which help to propel the cell in fluid environments.
- *Ciliates*: Ciliates have cilia, or hair-like structures, which line the cell. Cilia are used for movement, attachment, feeding and/or sensation.
- *Apicomplexa*: Apicomplexa are protozoa that are unique in their ability to produce spores. Apicomplexa are often pathogenic in humans and animals and are responsible for diseases such as malaria and toxoplasmosis.

Helminths

Helminths are parasitic worms, which can infect and cause disease in humans and animals. Helminths are multicellular, complex organisms that are visible to the human eye when they are mature. They produce eggs for reproduction and the eggs and larvae are then deposited by infected animals or people and penetrate their target host. Figure 2.3 shows the life cycle of the parasitic worm *Onchocerca volvulus* that causes onchocerciasis, also known as river blindness.

Many helminths are soil-transmitted. Their eggs are present in the faeces of people who are infected. These contaminate the soil in areas where sanitation is poor, which in turn contaminates food and water supplies. Soil-transmitted helminths can impair the nutritional status of their hosts, and can thus also impair physical and cognitive development among infected children. Soil-transmitted helminth infections are among the most common infections worldwide and affect the poorest and most deprived communities. It is estimated that more than 1.5 billion people, or 24% of the world's population, are infected with helminths. Most infectious diseases caused by helminths are restricted to tropical zones and primarily affect people who live in areas of poverty in low-income countries; the greatest number are found in sub-Saharan Africa, the Americas, China and East Asia (WHO, 2017).

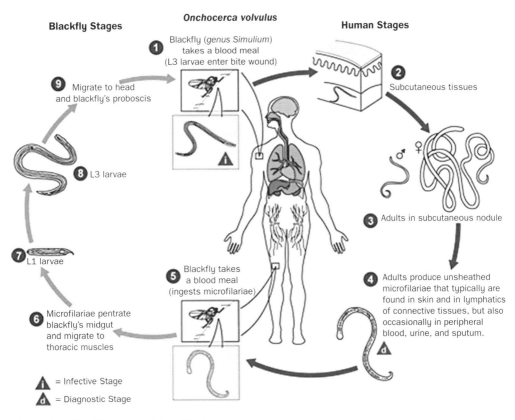

Blackfly Stages   *Onchocerca volvulus*   **Human Stages**

① Blackfly (*genus Simulium*)
  takes a blood meal
  (L3 larvae enter bite wound)

⑨ Migrate to head
  and blackfly's proboscis

② Subcutaneous tissues

⑧ L3 larvae

③ Adults in subcutaneous nodule

⑦ L1 larvae

⑤ Blackfly takes
  a blood meal
  (ingests microfilariae)

④ Adults produce unsheathed
  microfilariae that typically are
  found in skin and in lymphatics
  of connective tissues, but also
  occasionally in peripheral
  blood, urine, and sputum.

⑥ Microfilariae pentrate
  blackfly's midgut
  and migrate to
  thoracic muscles

▲i = Infective Stage
▲d = Diagnostic Stage

Figure 2.3 The life cycle of river blindness
Source: CDC, http://www.dpd.cdc.gov/dpdx/images/ParasiteImages/A-F/Filariasis/O_volvulus_LifeCycle.gi

The burden of disease caused by helminths is in general more associated with chronic, insidious morbidity, such as iron deficiency anaemia, than mortality. The burden of disease caused by helminths is substantial, yet the burden is not fully recognized, with inadequate resources dedicated to research, prevention and treatment. Many helminth diseases are often referred to as neglected tropical diseases.

There is no agreed taxonomy for helminths. They are usually grouped into the following three broad categories based mainly on their shared characteristics:

- Flatworms (platyhelminths), which cause diseases in humans, including schistosomiasis (bilhazia), fascioliasis and tapeworm infection.
- Thorny-headed worms (acanthocephalins), which do not usually cause infections in humans.
- Roundworms (nematodes), which cause diseases in humans, including ascariasis, dracunculiasis (guinea worm), elephantiasis, enterobiasis (pinworm), filariasis and hookworm infection.

Fungi

Fungi are plant-like organisms found naturally outdoors. There are more than 1.5 million species of fungus, of which only around 300 are responsible for illnesses in humans (CDC, 2014). Many fungal infections are relatively minor, commonly affecting the skin, nails and vagina. These include common fungal infections such as athlete's foot and ringworm. However, some are extremely serious and even life-threatening. For example, cryptococcal meningitis is a deadly brain infection caused by the soil-dwelling fungus *Cryptococcus*. Because fungi are common in the environment, people come into contact with fungal spores regularly, either by inhaling or touching them. Most of the time people do not get sick or, if they do, the infection is relatively minor. However, fungal infections are particularly dangerous to people who have weakened immune systems, such as those who have cancer or HIV.

Prevention of fungal infections is difficult, given the variety of environments that they can inhabit. There are some practical steps that can be taken in higher-risk settings, including maintenance of heating, ventilation and air-conditioning systems, which have been responsible for outbreaks of fungal diseases in healthcare facilities. Education for people at increased risk to encourage them to avoid exposure in certain settings is also important. Additional environmental considerations are given to construction activities, where certain moulds (for example, *Aspergillus*) can be disrupted and disseminated.

Prions

The discovery of prions as a type of infectious agent was relatively recent (Zabel and Reid, 2015). Before their discovery, researchers had believed that viruses were the smallest infectious agents. Prions are not living organisms. They are protein segments that fold in particular ways. When these protein segments are present in the brain, they interact with other proteins, stimulating a cascade of improper folding. At first glance, improperly folded proteins may not appear to be a significant threat. However, they cannot be broken down by normal mechanisms, leading to their accumulation in the brain. This accumulation can lead cells to malfunction and die, resulting in disease.

Prions are only responsible for a handful of human diseases, including: variant Creutzfeldt–Jakob disease (vCJD), also known as mad cow disease; fatal familial insomnia (FFI); Gertsmann-Straussler-Scheinker syndrome (GSS); kuru; and variably protease-sensitive prionopathy (VPSPr) (Prion Alliance, 2013). All of these diseases are very similar, with slight variations in the protein structure. Not all the diseases caused by prions are infectious. While some prions such as vCJD are transmitted, others can be genetic or they can develop spontaneously.

One of the many challenges associated with prions is that they cannot be eliminated from medical or surgical equipment through traditional sterilization practices. Most hospital-based sterilization practices target viruses and bacteria, with the aim of killing them and preventing secondary or iatrogenic transmission. Prions, not being alive, cannot be killed. In order to control prion infections, scientists have had to modify traditional techniques by increasing the intensity and duration of exposure to sterilizing agents, including heat (Rutala and Weber, 2010).

Parasites

A parasite is an organism that lives in or on another living thing. Parasites are not a distinct group of infectious agents. Some bacteria, viruses and protozoa and all helminths are parasites that can cause infectious disease. Typically, parasites derive their nutrients from their host, while either depleting the host's supply of nutrients or causing tissue damage. Parasites cause disease directly and indirectly through the toxins they produce. They can also act as the vectors of disease. Parasites come in many shapes and sizes, ranging from single-cell organisms, such as amoeba, to more complex multi-cell organisms. Parasites that live inside the body of the host are known as endoparasites. These include many helminths and protozoa. Parasites that live on the surface of the host are known as ectoparasites. These include lice, ticks and fleas.

Parasites are endemic the world over, with many people being infected for years without knowing. Depending on the parasite, people become infected in a number of ways. Infection can occur through exposure to contaminated soil, food or water; through vector transmission, including mosquitoes; and through contact with animals, such as domestic pets. Prevention of infection from parasites includes: proper treatment of water and sewage; limiting or enhancing the safety of exposure to animals; treating infections in humans and animals; and controlling the vectors of parasite transmission. Countries with more developed infrastructure have made significant advances in controlling many parasitic infections, particularly those that are spread through contaminated water or food. The greatest burden of disease from parasitic infection is experienced by the populations of low-income countries. However, certain parasitic diseases remain endemic in high- and middle-income countries, including Chagas disease, cysticercosis, toxocariasis, toxoplasmosis and trichomoniasis. People living in poor or disadvantaged communities are often most at risk.

Case study 2.2:   Malaria

Malaria is one of the best-known parasitic infections. In 2015, there were roughly 212 million malaria cases and an estimated 429,000 malaria deaths (WHO, 2016a).

Malaria is caused by the protozoan parasite *Plasmodium*. There are over 100 known species of *Plasmodium*, but only five species are capable of infecting humans and causing disease. These are:

- *P. falciparum*: one of the more virulent strains of *Plasmodium*, which is found predominantly in tropical areas of sub-Saharan Africa.
- *P. vivax*: found predominantly in Asia and Latin America and capable of re-emerging after a period of latency.
- *P. ovale*: found predominantly in West Africa.
- *P. malariae*: has a worldwide distribution and capable of developing into a chronic infection.
- *P. knowlesi*: naturally infects macaques and has recently been recognized to be a cause of zoonotic malaria in humans in Southeast Asia. It can progress rapidly from initial infection to fulminant disease (CDC, 2015).

The *Plasmodium* parasites are transmitted via the bite of female *Anopheles* mosquitoes, from reservoirs that may be humans or animals, to the susceptible hosts, which may also be humans or animals. The mosquitoes are not reservoirs of infection, but rather vehicles to transmit the parasites from one source to another. For this reason, they are referred to as 'vectors'. Once released into the bloodstream of a host, the *Plasmodium* parasites first infect cells of the liver, where reproduction intensifies. Eventually, the parasites enter the blood, attacking red blood cells and targeting blood vessels and various organs, including the spleen, brain and bone marrow. The infected person becomes ill as tissues are damaged, resulting in flu-like symptoms, respiratory distress, pain and even death.

 Activity 2.2

Based on your reading so far, what measures can you think of to control malaria? How do they work to control the disease? Do you think they work by changing factors related to the host, the agent or the environment?

Feedback

Measures you might have suggested include:

- *Insecticide-treated mosquito nets*: such nets work by reducing the exposure of the host (the individual person) to the vector (mosquitoes) that transmits the infectious agent (plasmodia).
- *Spraying mosquito-infested areas and indoor residual spraying*: works by reducing the number of vectors (mosquitoes) that transmit the infectious agent (plasmodia).

- *Insect repellent*: works by reducing the exposure of the host (the individual person) to the vector (mosquitoes) that transmits the infectious agent (plasmodia).
- *Malaria prophylaxis*: works by killing the infectious agent (plasmodia) when they have entered the host's body (the individual) before they can cause disease.
- *Ensuring the provision of diagnostic and treatment services*: reduces disease and prevents deaths and can also contribute to reducing malaria cases by reducing the number of people who can transmit the infection to others. The best available treatment, particularly for *P. falciparum* malaria, is artemisinin-based combination therapy (ACT) (WHO, 2016a).
- *Programmes to reduce malnutrition*: work by reducing the susceptibility of the host (the individual) by improving their immunity.

Microorganisms

Many infectious agents are microorganisms. A microorganism is an extremely small living form that can only be seen using a microscope, as it is not visible to the naked eye. The word microbe is often used interchangeably with microorganism. Microorganisms, or microbes, may be single-celled or multicellular. Microorganisms are very diverse and include different types of infectious agents, including all bacteria, most protozoa and some species of fungi. There is ongoing debate as to whether viruses constitute microorganism or are organic structures that interact with living organisms (Villarreal, 2008).

Microorganisms perform a wide variety of functions, ranging from recycling organic material into usable soil, through to creating and regulating gases, digestion and metabolism. Microorganisms also appear to play an important role in the evolution of life (Brucker and Bordenstein, 2013). While it is true that certain microorganisms do cause disease, and this has been the focus of much of medicine, most interactions with microorganisms do not. Research suggests that there are likely to be 10 million trillion microbes on Earth for every single human being (Lougheed, 2012). Scientific understanding of microorganisms is developing all the time, with new advances providing insights with many applications, including improving health.

Host

Infectious diseases are caused by pathogens that spread from person to person, either directly or indirectly. The mechanism by which an infectious disease is spread is known as a mode of transmission. We discuss modes of transmission in the following chapter. While transmission requires some form of exposure to an infectious agent, exposure in itself does not guarantee that an individual will become infected. As this chapter has already discussed, humans are exposed to many infectious agents that are present in and on the human body and in the environment, but they do not develop infectious disease. Infection occurs when a pathogen has the opportunity to invade an individual. Whether there is such an opportunity is influenced by many factors, including level of exposure and the suscep-tibility of that individual to infection, known as host susceptibility. There are a number of factors that affect exposure and host susceptibility, and these will now be discussed.

Immunity

The function of the immune system is to protect the body against all disease threats. The immune system does not only respond to potential threats from infectious agents, it responds to *any* cells or foreign bodies that are perceived to be a risk. This includes rapidly dividing, cancerous cells, which the body will attempt to eliminate in an effort to maintain balance. The mechanisms used by the immune system to protect the body from perceived and actual threats are extremely complex. There is a scientific specialism dedicated to the study of the immune system known as immunology. This section now presents a broad outline of immune functioning to enable the reader to understand better the relationship between pathogens, immunity, infection and disease.

Innate immunity

Innate immunity refers to a range of mechanisms that the body uses to defend itself by preventing the introduction of infectious agents and the spread of infection or disease. Innate immunity differs from adaptive immunity in that adaptive immunity results from previous exposure, including immunization, and is specific to certain infectious agents. Features of the innate immune system include anatomical barriers, inflammation, the complement system and cell-mediated immunity. These features are described below.

Anatomical barriers: One of the most potent aspects of the immune system is the skin. This organ protects other sensitive organs inside the body and helps to maintain homeostasis, or balance within the body. The skin is frequently colonized with a wide range of microorganisms, which in general pose little threat as long as they are maintained on the outside of the skin. Only a few pathogens, such as some parasitic worms, are able to penetrate through skin. Other anatomical barriers of note include hair, such as the hair lining the nose. These hairs act as filters that prevent larger particles from entering the body through respiratory passages.

Inflammation: Once a pathogen or another foreign body enters the body, one of the first responses is the acute inflammatory process, which forms part of the innate immune system. Certain cells, when damaged either by physical trauma or through infection, initiate a process of inflammation by stimulating the release of inflammatory mediators. The inflammatory process enables immune cells to reach the site of trauma or pathogenic invasion as blood vessels dilate. The inflammation of tissue also creates a physical barrier to prevent invading organisms spreading systemically. The inflammatory process happens rapidly and is time-limited, with inflammation only lasting for as long as the threat is perceived to be present.

Complement system: The complement system literally 'complements' the work of other immune processes. When tissue damage occurs through trauma or other means, the complement system is activated and initiates a biological response to infection involving protein production. These complement proteins signal other immune cells to travel to the site of inflammation. They also help in identifying target cells for destruction, or attack the cells directly. The complement system, like inflammation, is a rapid response against perceived threats to the body.

Cellular immunity: Cellular immunity involves a group of cells in the body that help fight infection by identifying non-specific threats and responding. Once stimulated, these immune cells arrive at the scene of invasion and begin targeting, engulfing or destroying pathogenic cells. They also destroy normal cells that have been invaded by material identified as being foreign.

Innate immunity provides an essential primary response to any organism or tissue perceived as being foreign and strives to prevent the progression of infections that people have not previously encountered. Many symptoms commonly associated with infection and illness, such as inflammation, fever and pain, are in fact the direct result of the innate immune system's response to prevent the development and spread of infection.

Adaptive immunity

When an individual is exposed to a pathogen, the body learns to recognize that specific pathogen, so that it can mount a comprehensive and rapid response to it in the future. Adaptive immunity develops throughout a person's life as they recover from infection with particular pathogens, or through immunization. Immunization is the process of making a person immune to a pathogen by exposing them to that pathogen, usually through the administration of a vaccine. When a person has not come into contact with a particular pathogen before, they are called *immunologically naïve* to that pathogen or its related disease.

The part of a pathogen that produces an immune response is known as an *antigen*. When the pathogen enters the body a second time, the antigen triggers circulating antibodies, which are specific to it. These antibodies either destroy the pathogen directly or they activate the complement system, thus attracting other immune cells with the capacity to neutralize the pathogen.

The advantage of adaptive immunity is that it is highly adapted to address specific threats. This means that the pathogen has very little opportunity to avoid the immune system's response and that the response itself is tailored to the specific pathogen and so will be much more effective.

Case study 2.3:   Influenza

Influenza, known more commonly as flu, is an infectious disease caused by a virus. It is spread by respiratory or contact transmission. It primarily affects the respiratory system. Influenza is associated with significant morbidity and mortality every year, especially among vulnerable groups such as children, older people and people with reduced immunity. For this reason, immunization against influenza for vulnerable groups is recommended by the World Health Organization (WHO) and is widespread in many countries. However, there are many different strains of influenza and the virus mutates frequently. This means when the viral strain is new, people do not have underlying immunity from earlier vaccination or infection. Every year, the WHO predicts which strains of the virus are most likely to be circulating in the following year. Influenza vaccines can be attenuated live vaccines, which means they are alive but weakened so they cannot cause infection, or inactivated, which means that only the dead virus particle is included in the vaccine. Once injected into the body, the vaccine is recognized as being foreign. This recognition triggers an immediate inflammatory reaction and other innate immune responses. After this initial exposure, the body begins to produce antibodies specific to the pathogen it encountered, the particular strain of influenza. If the antigen associated with this strain of influenza presents again, the response will be much more rapid and robust, thus minimizing the degree of illness experienced by the individual. If a person is immunologically naïve to that strain of influenza – that is, they have not been infected with or vaccinated against the same (or a similar) strain – their body will not recognize the antigen and will not have developed antibodies. They are far more likely to experience prolonged and severe symptoms, and possibly complications leading to death.

Lifestyle

Lifestyle and, more specifically, certain risk-related behaviours will influence an individual's risk for contracting an infection and developing disease. This is because lifestyle can increase or decrease a person's level of exposure to an infectious agent. For example, people who inject drugs are more likely to get blood-borne infectious diseases such as hepatitis C or HIV.

In addition, lifestyle can impact on susceptibility. For example, there is evidence that smoking increases the risk of tuberculosis (TB) in people who are exposed to the bacterium (US Department of Health and Human Services, 2014).

Health status

A person's overall health status plays a major role in susceptibility to various infections. Health status includes functioning, fitness, physical illness, weight, nutritional status and mental wellbeing. People with a good health status have more effective immune systems that are better able to fight infection. Being infected with one pathogen often predisposes people to other infections, and the development of disease. Some diseases are particularly harmful to the immune system. For example, people who have HIV are 20–30 times more likely than people who do not to develop TB (University of California San Francisco, 2013).

Nutrition

Good nutrition is essential in ensuring optimal health, and also in preventing the onset of infections and disease. Malnutrition or under-nutrition is associated with increased risk of mortality from infectious disease, particularly among children (Rice et al., 2000). It puts children at greater risk of dying from common infections, increases the frequency and severity of such infections, and contributes to delayed recovery. In addition, the interaction between under-nutrition and infection can create a potentially lethal cycle of worsening illness and deteriorating nutritional status. Nearly half of all deaths in children under 5 years old are attributable to malnutrition or under-nutrition and it is widespread in Africa and Asia (UNICEF, 2016). This translates into the unnecessary loss of about 3 million young lives a year.

The problem of under-nutrition is not exclusively a problem of access to, or the availability of, adequate food supplies. Anorexia nervosa is a condition in which people restrict their food intake significantly, and often reduce their weight to dangerously low levels. Anorexia nervosa has been associated with many serious and harmful side-effects, one of which is vulnerability to infections. The poor nutritional status of people living with anorexia nervosa typically leads to an impaired formation of immune cells, which in turn increases vulnerability to infectious disease (Devuyst et al., 1993).

In addition to under-nutrition, poor nutrition and obesity also increase vulnerability to infection. Sub-standard nutrition, including unbalanced diets that lack essential nutrients, impacts on the immune system. There is also strong evidence indicating that obesity negatively impacts on the immune system (Milner and Beck, 2012). Obesity is recognized as a major public health problem. In 2014, over 600 million adults were obese (WHO, 2016b). Although this was once considered a high-income country problem, it is now increasing in low- and middle-income countries, particularly in urban settings. As with many of the other factors influencing vulnerability to infection, people living in poverty often are at a higher risk of poor nutritional status.

Psychological wellbeing

Psychological wellbeing can influence susceptibility to infection through a number of pathways. There is evidence that some groups of people with depression are more likely to engage in risk-taking behaviour, for example having multiple sexual partners (Langille et al., 2011). These behaviours increase the likelihood of exposure to a pathogen, and influence susceptibility (Khan et al., 2009). There is also emerging evidence of the relationship between depression and the down-regulation of immune functioning (Kiecolt-Glaser and Glaser, 2002).

Genetics

Genes are a set of instructions for the growth and development of every cell in the body. Genes are inherited but are also influenced by the environment. For example, a person may inherit genes for being tall, but if their diet does not provide them with the necessary nutrients, they may not grow very tall. Genes can influence an individual's susceptibility to infection by determining cellular and adaptive immunity. For example, the majority of people are vulnerable to infection with HIV, but this is not universally true. There are some people who, through their history of exposure and lifestyle, would be expected to have become HIV-positive but have not. Distinct genetic characteristics have made these people resistant to HIV infection, despite repeated exposures (Pancino et al., 2010). With more research, it may be possible to develop treatments and vaccines based on natural genetic resistance to HIV and other infections.

Microbiota

Microbiota is the ecology of microorganisms that live inside and on the surface of the body. There is growing evidence that microbiota play a role in resisting certain infections and maintaining balance in the body. The immune system's development is shaped by microbiota. The immune system in turn influences microbiota (Cahenzli et al., 2013). The adequate presence and balanced makeup of microbiota is essential to ensure that no particular microorganism becomes dominant and potentially problematic. For example, Clostridium difficile is a microorganism commonly found in the intestines of humans. When people are treated with certain antibiotics, they kill much of the natural microbiota in the intestines, but often not *Clostridium difficile* that has developed natural resistance to powerful antibiotics. Because microbiota play a key role in keeping *Clostridium difficile* in check, these bacteria can then become dominant, leading to infection and disease. There is growing interest among scientists and researchers about the role played by microbiota in resisting infection and how it interacts with the immune system (Garrett, 2017).

Environment

Environment is the third part of the epidemiological triad that describes the causation of infectious diseases. Environment includes external factors that affect both the infectious agent and the host. These are made up of physical factors, such as geology, geography and climate. As this chapter has already explained, some infectious diseases are more common in tropical areas because the infectious agents and their vectors thrive there. Agricultural practices and large infrastructure projects, such as dams, can cause changes in the environment that result in the introduction or increase of infectious agents. Environmental factors that impact on communicable diseases are discussed in more detail in Chapter 11 of this book and in *Environment, Health and Sustainable Development* (Hutchinson and Kovats, 2017), which is part of the Understanding Public Health series.

There is also a range of social and economic circumstances that impact upon infectious agents and hosts. These are termed the social determinants of health. They are the conditions in which people are born, grow up, live, work and age (Morgan and Cragg, 2013). These can include, but are not restricted to: education, employment, income, crime, physical environments, housing and essential services. Populations living in temporary or sub-standard housing, for example, might not have access to clean water or sanitation, thereby being more vulnerable to water-borne infections. The social determinants of health influence infectious disease in a number of ways. First, they impact on whether a person has the means to access the essential requirements for healthy living such as good nutrition and housing, which impact on immune function and susceptibility to infection. Second, they determine the general availability in a population of proper sanitation, hygiene and clean water, which are essential to prevent infectious agents rapidly spreading and causing disease. Third, lifestyle and behavioural factors associated with health and ill health are strongly influenced by the social determinants of health. For example, the likelihood that an individual will start smoking is heavily influenced by the social determinants of health. Lifestyle and behaviour impact on exposure to infectious agents and host susceptibility. Fourth, the social determinants of health contribute to psychological wellbeing, which, as discussed above, impacts on susceptibility to infectious disease.

Identify a policy or project that seeks to influence the social determinants of health in your country. Describe how this will impact on communicable diseases.

Feedback

You may have identified projects on the social determinants of health, including those related to infrastructure, employment, housing, income, education, gender equality, the built environment and access to services. You may have suggested that these could result in improvements in educational achievement or levels of unemployment, which means that individuals are likely to experience better overall health, for example through nutrition and exercise. This may improve their immunity. You may have suggested improved infrastructure that will reduce reservoirs and prevent the spread of infectious agents in communities, neighbourhoods or cities, such as sewage treatment and water provision. You may also have suggested interventions that help people to reduce their own exposure to infectious agents, such as policies on gender empowerment that better enable women to refuse unprotected sex.

Marginalization

Marginalization refers to the process by which groups of people experience disadvantage and discrimination because of characteristics including gender, gender identity, age, ethnicity, religion or belief, disability, sexual orientation, education, employment status, income, or where they live. People who are part of marginalized groups may be deprived of educational and employment opportunities, be denied legal and political rights, and have difficult accessing services, including health services. While being marginalized does not necessarily mean that a group is more vulnerable to communicable disease, being marginalized can be a significant cause of this vulnerability. This is because marginalization can impact on all three elements of the epidemiological triad. For example, marginalized groups who are forcibly displaced due to violence or persecution may be exposed to infectious *agents* that they would not have ordinarily been exposed to and have no immunity to as they move to new geographical locations. People who are members of marginalized groups may have increased *host* susceptibility to infectious agents because they have poor health and nutritional status due to precarious employment and low income. They may also have difficult accessing health services, including vaccination programmes. Finally, they may be exposed to *environments* that contribute to the spread of communicable disease, such as poor quality, overcrowded housing.

Summary

This chapter has provided an overview of how infectious agents, hosts and environmental factors interact to cause infectious disease. It briefly described the main types of infectious agents, namely: bacteria, viruses, protozoa, helminths, fungi and prions. Many of these infectious agents are microorganisms, but microorganisms also exist in huge numbers on and inside the human body and in the environment, and the vast majority do not cause infectious disease. The chapter also addressed some of the main factors that influence whether a person is likely to become infected and develop an infectious disease. Finally, the chapter provided a brief overview of environmental factors that influence infectious agents and hosts. Understanding this interaction of agent, host and environment is important in developing and implementing effective control measure for communicable diseases.

Further reading

Hutchinson, E. and Kovats, S. (2017) *Environment, Health and Sustainable Development*, 2nd edn. London: Open University Press.

References

Barrett, S. (2004) Eradication vs. control: the economics of global infectious disease policy, *Bulletin of the World Health Organization*, 82 (9): 683–688.

Brucker, R.M. and Bordenstein, S.R. (2013) The hologenomic basis of speciation: gut bacteria cause hybrid lethality in the genus *Nasonia*, *Science*, 341 (6146): 667–669.

Cahenzli, J., Balmer, M.L. and McCoy, K.D. (2013) Microbial-immune cross-talk and regulation of the immune system, *Immunology*, 138: 12–22.

Centers for Disease Control and Prevention (CDC) (2014) *Types of fungal diseases*. Available at: http://www.cdc.gov/fungal/diseases/index.html [accessed 30 January 2017].

Centers for Disease Control and Prevention (CDC) (2015) *Malaria parasites*. Available at: http://www.cdc.gov/malaria/about/biology/parasites.html [accessed 30 November 2015].

Devuyst, O., Lambert, M., Rodhain, J., Lefebvre, C. and Coche, E. (1993) Haematological changes and infectious complications in anorexia nervosa: a case-control study, *QJM: An International Journal of Medicine*, 86 (12): 791–799.

Diehl, W.E., Patel, N., Halm, K. and Johnson, W.E. (2016) Tracking interspecies transmission and long-term evolution of an ancient retrovirus using the genomes of modern mammals, *eLife*, 5: e12704.

Garrett, W.S. (2017) Gut microbiota in 2016: a banner year for gut microbiota research, *Nature Reviews Gastroenterology and Hepatology*, 14 (2): 78–80.

Hutchinson, E. and Kovats, S. (2017) *Environment, Health and Sustainable Development*, 2nd edn. London: Open University Press.

Janeway, C.A., Jr., Travers, P., Walport, M. and Schlomchik, M.J. (2001) *Immunobiology: The Immune System in Health and Disease*, 5th edn. New York: Garland Publishing.

Khan, M.R., Kaufman, J.S., Pence, B.W., Gaynes, B.N., Adimora, A.A., Weir, S.S. *et al.* (2009) Depression, sexually transmitted infection, and sexual risk behavior among young adults in the United States, *Archives of Pediatrics and Adolescent Medicine*, 163 (7): 644–652.

Kiecolt-Glaser, J.K. and Glaser, R. (2002) Depression and immune function: central pathways to morbidity and mortality, *Journal of Psychosomatic Research*, 53 (4): 873–876.

Langille, D., Asbridge, M., Kisely, S. and Wilson, K. (2011) Risk of depression and multiple sexual risk-taking behaviours in adolescents in Nova Scotia, Canada, *Sexual Health*, 9: 254–260.

Lougheed, K. (2012) There are fewer microbes out there than you think, *Nature,* 27 August.

Milner, J.J. and Beck, M.A. (2012) The impact of obesity on the immune response to infection, *Proceedings of the Nutrition Society*, 71 (2): 298–306. Available at: http://doi.org/10.1017/S0029665112000158.

Morgan, M. and Cragg, L. (2013) The determinants of health, in L. Cragg, M. Davies and W. Macdowall (eds.) *Health Promotion Theory*, 2nd edn. (pp. 98–113). Maidenhead: Open University Press.

Pancino, G., Saez-Cirion, A., Scott-Algara, D. and Paul, P. (2010) Natural resistance to HIV infection: lessons learned from HIV-exposed uninfected individuals, *Journal of Infectious Diseases*, 202 (suppl. 3): S345–S350.

Prion Alliance (2013) *What are human prion diseases?* Available at: http://www.prionalliance.org/2013/12/02/what-are-human-prion-diseases/ [accessed 30 January 2017].

Rice, A.L., Sacco, L., Hyder, A. and Black, R.E. (2000) Malnutrition as an underlying cause of childhood deaths associated with infectious diseases in developing countries, *Bulletin of the World Health Organization*, 78 (10): 1207–1221.

Rutala, W.A. and Weber, D.J. (2010) Guideline for disinfection and sterilization of prion-contaminated medical instruments, *Infection Control*, 31 (2): 107–117.

Sender, R., Fuchs, S. and Milo, R. (2016) Revised estimates for the number of human and bacteria cells in the body, *PLoS Biology*, 14 (8): e1002533.

Sze, D.Y., Reid, T.R. and Rose, S.C. (2013) Oncolytic virotherapy, *Journal of Vascular and Interventional Radiology*, 24 (8): 1115–1122.

Talaro, K.P. and Chess, B. (2014) *Foundations in Microbiology*, 9th edn. New York: McGraw-Hill Education.

UNICEF (2016) *Malnutrition: Current status and progress*. Available at: http://data.unicef.org/topic/nutrition/malnutrition/.

University of California San Francisco (2013) Tuberculosis and HIV, *HIV InSite*. Available at: http://hivinsite.ucsf.edu/InSite?page=kb-05-01-06 [accessed 30 November 2015].

US Department of Health and Human Services (2014) *The health consequences of smoking – 50 years of progress: A report of the Surgeon General, 2014*. Atlanta, GA: US Department of Health and Human Services.

Villarreal, L.P. (2008) Are viruses alive?, *Scientific American*, 291: 100–105.

World Health Organization (WHO) (2016a) *10 facts on malaria*. Geneva: WHO. Available at: http://www.who.int/features/factfiles/malaria/en/ [accessed 30 January 2017].

World Health Organization (WHO) (2016b) *Factsheet on obesity and overweight*. Geneva: WHO. Available at: http://www.who.int/mediacentre/factsheets/fs311/en [accessed 30 January 2017].

World Health Organization (WHO) (2017) *Soil-transmitted helminth infections*. Available at: http://www.who.int/mediacentre/factsheets/fs366/en/ [accessed 30 January 2017].

Zabel, M.D. and Reid, C. (2015) A brief history of prions, *Pathogens and Disease*, 73 (9): ftv087.

The chain of infection and modes of transmission

3

Liza Cragg

Overview

The previous chapter explained how agent, host and environment interact to cause communicable disease. This chapter explores the chain of infection whereby an infectious agent enters a susceptible host. It describes places where infectious agents live and multiply, known as reservoirs. It then explains the different ways an infectious agent can enter a susceptible host. These are known as modes of transmission. Understanding how a communicable disease is transmitted, or spread, is an important step in developing effective measures to control it.

Learning objectives

After reading this chapter, you will be able to:

- describe the chain of infection
- understand the importance of reservoirs in infectious diseases control
- describe the main portals of exit and entry
- explain the modes of transmission by which communicable disease is spread

Key terms

Chronic carriers: People who carry an infectious agent for an extended period, usually defined as longer than 6 or 12 months depending on the pathogen, without displaying, or after recovering from, signs of the disease.

Convalescent carriers: People who have recovered from a disease but are still carrying the infectious agent and able to transmit it.

Fomite: An inanimate (non-living) object that can carry an infectious agent in indirect contact transmission.

Inapparent infection: People who do not develop any symptoms as a result of infection or whose symptoms are so mild they do not notice them.

Incubation period: The period of time between exposure to an infectious agent and onset of clinical symptoms.

Incubatory carriers: People who are infected and will become ill but have not yet started to show symptoms, although they are already able to transmit the disease to another person.

Infectious period: The time period during which infected individuals are able to transmit an infectious agent to other susceptible hosts or vectors.

Latent period: The period of time between exposure to an infectious agent and onset of the infectious period.

Transmissibility: The ability of a pathogen to be passed from one host to another.

Vector: Any living organism that transfers an infectious agent from one host to another.

Zoonoses or zoonotic diseases: Infections that are naturally transmissible from vertebrate animals to humans and vice versa.

The chain of infection

Transmission can be defined as is the process by which an infectious agent passes from an infected host to a susceptible host. The ability of an infectious agent to do this is referred to as its transmissibility. Transmission requires the infectious agent to leave the infected host from a portal of exit, and enter the susceptible host though a portal of entry. The different mechanisms an infectious agent can use to do this are known as modes of transmission. The sequence of events involved in the transmission process is sometimes referred to as the chain of infection, as described in Figure 3.1. This chain involves the following six links:

1. An infectious agent
2. A reservoir
3. A portal of exit
4. A mode of transmission
5. A portal of entry
6. A susceptible host.

RESERVOIR   MODE OF TRANSMISSION   SUSCEPTIBLE HOST

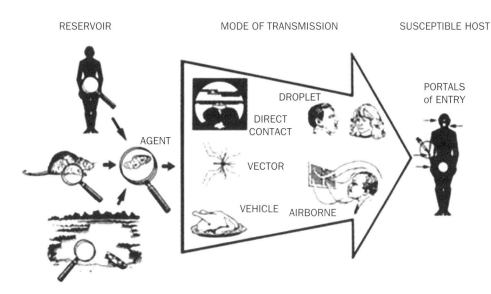

Figure 3.1 The chain of infection

Source: Centers for Disease Control and Prevention (1992) *Principles of Epidemiology,* 2nd edn. Atlanta, GA: US Department of Health and Human Services, https://www.cdc.gov/ophss/csels/dsepd/ss1978/lesson1/section10.html.

Controlling a communicable disease requires breaking this chain of infection. This involves interventions that:

- eliminate or reduce the infectious agent that causes the disease, such as through treatment of infected people or animals that act as reservoirs, and environmental improvements;
- prevent the infectious agent entering new susceptible hosts by stopping transmission, such as through the use of condoms to protect against sexually transmitted diseases;
- reduce the susceptibility of potential hosts, such as vaccination campaigns.

The previous chapter explained the different types of infectious agent and factors that determine host susceptibility. This chapter explains the other links in the chain of infection: reservoirs, portals of exit, portals of entry and modes of transmission. Developing the right type and combination of interventions requires a good understanding of these as they relate to the infectious agent responsible for each communicable disease.

Reservoirs

A reservoir is a location where an infectious agent can survive and multiply. As explained in Chapter 2, there are different potential reservoirs, depending on the particular infectious agent. Some infectious agents can survive in more than one type of reservoir. Understanding what the potential reservoirs are for a particular disease is important for designing effective control measures. However, in some cases reservoirs for infectious diseases, particularly new and emerging ones, cannot be identified with certainty (Hayden, 2002). An infectious disease that has an unidentified reservoir can be difficult to control because it is not possible to eliminate or reduce the infectious agents that cause the disease. Reservoirs fall into three groups, which will now be described: human reservoirs, animal reservoirs and environmental reservoirs.

Human reservoirs

Humans are often the main reservoir for infectious diseases that affect humans. For some of these diseases, such as measles, the infected person, who is the reservoir, transmits the disease directly to another person. For other diseases, such as malaria, a vector is required for transmission. Modes of transmission are discussed later in this chapter.

Infected humans can be divided into two types: people with symptoms and people without symptoms. People with symptoms, often referred to acute clinical cases, are people who have become ill as a result of their infection. People without symptoms are those who are infected but have not become unwell, often referred to as asymptomatic cases. Different infectious diseases result in different types of asymptomatic cases.

Asymptomatic cases include incubatory carriers, who are people that are infected and will become ill but have not yet started to show symptoms, although they are already able to transmit the disease to another person. For example, the incubation period for hepatitis B averages 6 weeks but may be as long as 6 months. Asymptomatic cases also include people with inapparent infections, who do not develop any symptoms or whose symptoms are so mild they do not notice them. For example, as many as half of all dengue-infected individuals have no clinical signs or symptoms of disease. Convalescent carriers, defined as people who have recovered from a disease but are still carrying the infectious agent and able to transmit it, are another type of asymptomatic case. For example, people who have had cholera can continue to excrete the bacteria in their faeces for several months after they have recovered. Finally, asymptomatic cases also include chronic carriers who are people that continue to carry an infectious agent for an extended period (usually defined as longer than 6 or 12 months depending on the pathogen) without displaying, or after recovering from, clinical signs or symptoms of the disease. For example, between 1% and 5% of patients with typhoid fever, depending on age, become chronic carriers harbouring *Salmonella typhi* in the gallbladder (WHO, 2011).

Communicable diseases that only have human reservoirs are generally easier to control or eradicate completely than those that also have animal and/or environmental reservoirs. This is because it may be feasible to identify and target all reservoirs to prevent the infectious agents being transmitted. However, communicable diseases which often lead to asymptomatic carrier states in infected hosts are generally more problematic to control than those for which asymptomatic states are less common and/or less prolonged. This is because people with symptoms are likely to seek care, be diagnosed and be treated, which eliminates or reduces the infectious agent they carry, preventing them from transmitting it to others. In addition, when people are ill their activities and interactions with other people are likely to reduce, so they are less likely to infect others. However, people who are asymptomatic often do not know they are infected and so do not seek treatment or change their behaviour to avoid transmitting the infection to others.

Animal reservoirs

Humans can also be infected by diseases that have animal reservoirs. An infection that is naturally transmissible from vertebrate animals to humans and vice versa is known as a zoonosis. One literature review identified that 61% of 1415 species of infectious organisms known to be pathogenic to humans are zoonotic (Taylor *et al.*, 2001). As with human reservoirs, animals can carry and transmit certain pathogens to humans or other animals, but not develop disease themselves. Some zoonoses are known to have affected humans for centuries. Examples include plague, which comes from rats, and rabies, which comes from mammals. Many of the important infectious diseases affecting humans that have emerged recently, such as human immunodeficiency virus (HIV) and Ebola virus disease (EVD), are thought to be zoonoses. Research suggests that zoonoses may be an increasingly important source of emerging infectious diseases, with one study finding that 60% of emerging infectious diseases are zoonotic (Jones *et al.*, 2008). The factors that drive the emergence of zoonotic diseases are complex and include ecological, political, economic and social forces (National Research Council, 2009).

Growing recognition of the importance of zoonoses to human health has led to the development of a new paradigm known as One Health, which emphasizes the critical connections between animal health, human health and the environment. The aim of One Health is 'To improve health and well-being through the prevention of risks and the mitigation of effects of crises that originate at the interface between humans, animals and their various environments' (One Health, 2017). It advocates integrated approaches as a means to improve human, animal and environmental health. Integrated in this context means multidisciplinary, cross-sectoral and cross-level approaches designed to reduce and address health risks (Zinsstag *et al.*, 2011). One Health is generating closer collaboration between human, animal and environmental health specialists and researchers, which is becoming critically important in an era of rapid and profound anthropogenic changes, including climate change. The impacts of climate change on communicable diseases are discussed in more detail in Chapter 11 of this book and in *Environment, Health and Sustainable Development* (Hutchinson and Kovats, 2017), which is part of the Understanding Public Health series.

Environmental reservoirs

Water and the soil are common environmental reservoirs for infectious diseases. Water is a reservoir of many bacteria, including *Vibrio cholerae*, which causes the acute and potentially fatal diarrhoeal disease cholera. Many types of fungi that cause infectious disease live and multiply in soil. Air conditioning and air-cooling systems are also an environmental reservoir for some infectious agents, including the bacteria that cause Legionnaires' disease, *Legionella pneumophila*.

Portal of exit

After the reservoir, the next link in the chain of infection is the portal of exit. This is the means by which the infectious agent leaves the reservoir. Some infectious agents have only one portal of exit but others have several different ones. The portal of exit in human or animal reservoirs is often close to where the symptoms of the diseases are experienced. For example, the portal of exit for cholera is in faeces; for rhinovirus and influenza viruses it is the respiratory tract; and for scabies it is skin lesions. The most common portals for infectious diseases in humans and animals are:

- the respiratory system, in droplets expressed by sneezing, coughing and spitting;
- the genitourinary organs, in urine or sexual fluids;
- the digestive system, through the mouth or faeces;
- the skin, in lesions or insect bites;
- the placenta, from mother to foetus.

Portal of entry

The portal of entry needs to give the infectious agent access to an environment in which it can live and multiply. Sometimes the entry portal into a new host is the same as the exit portal. For example, rhinovirus can exit and enter through the respiratory system via the nose and mouth. Alternatively, an infectious agent may enter through a different portal than that which it uses to exit. For example, infectious agents that are transmitted through the faecal–oral route exit the source host in faeces from the anus and enter the new host through the mouth. The portal of entry of an infectious agent is linked to its mode of transmission. These modes and their respective portals of entry are discussed below. This section briefly describes the main portals of entry and their key features.

Figure 3.2 shows the main portals of entry infectious agents use to enter humans. The largest potential portal of entry is the skin. However, as discussed in Chapter 2, the skin is well adapted to protect against infections. It is covered with an outer layer of cells that act as a barrier. Infectious agents enter where the skin is breached, through an insect bite or a cut. Some infectious agents, such as the cercariae (the infectious larval stage) of schistosomes, are even able to penetrate unbroken skin. Where the portal of entry is through the nose, the mouth or the genital area, the infectious agent enters the body via the mucous membranes. Mucous membranes are moist linings of body passages and internal cavities involved in the absorption and secretion of substances. The mucous membranes are not covered with the same barrier cells as the skin, as this would hinder their function. When infectious agents enter the mouth, they can also reach the digestive system. The chemicals involved in digestion kill many infectious agents but some are resistant. More rarely, some infectious agents, such as measles, can enter the body through the conjunctiva of

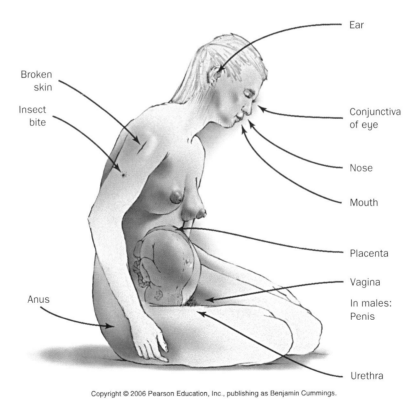

Copyright © 2006 Pearson Education, Inc., publishing as Benjamin Cummings.

Figure 3.2 The main portals of entry for infectious agents

Source: Bauman, Robert W., Microbiology with Diseases by Taxonomy: International Edition, 2nd Ed., © 2007. Reprinted by permission of Pearson Education, Inc., New York.

the eyes. The placenta can also act as a portal of entry for an infectious agent to be transmitted from mother to child. This is known as vertical transmission.

Modes of transmission

A mode of transmission is how an infectious agent leaves the portal of exit and reaches the portal of entry.

 Activity 3.1

Return to the list you made for Activity 2.1 of the different communicable diseases that you have been affected by. Based on your reading so far, how do you think these were transmitted?

Feedback

Modes of transmission are summarized in Table 3.1 and described in more detail next.

The main modes of transmission for communicable diseases can be divided into two groups: contact and non-contact. Many communicable diseases are able to use multiple modes of transmission, for example measles can be spread by indirect, droplet and respiratory transmission. In addition, the relative importance of different modes can change, with infectious agents having the potential to shift mode of transmission in response to selective pressures, including disease control interventions (Webster *et al.*, 2017). Each mode of transmission is summarized in Table 3.1 and described below.

Table 3.1 Summary of the main modes of transmission for communicable disease

	Direct	Direct physical contact between an infected person or animal and a susceptible host, including touching, kissing and sexual intercourse. Examples include HIV, influenza and chlamydia.
Contact	Indirect	An infectious agent is left on an object (referred to in this context as a 'fomite') by an infected person or animal and is then transferred to a susceptible host who subsequently touches the object. Examples include rhinovirus and methicillin-resistant *Staphylococcus aureus* (MRSA).
	Droplet	Droplets are projected by an infected person sneezing, coughing, speaking or spitting that then reach a susceptible host. Examples include influenza and rhinovirus.

	Airborne	Infectious agents are carried by dust or droplet nuclei suspended in air. These are very small and can remain suspended for some time, compared with droplets that fall to the ground within a metre or so. These are then inhaled by susceptible hosts. Examples include measles, chickenpox and tuberculosis (TB).
Non-contact	Vector-borne	Vectors are small animals, such as mosquitoes and ticks that carry infectious agents from a reservoir or host to a susceptible host. Examples include malaria, visceral leishmaniasis and plague.
	Vehicle-borne	Inanimate objects or biological products, including food and water that carry infectious agents. Examples include cholera and hepatitis A.

Contact transmission: direct

Direct contact transmission involves physical contact between an infected person (or animal) and a potential susceptible host. The infectious agent is transmitted in the bodily fluids of the infected person, which include blood, semen and vaginal secretions.

Sexual transmission is one of the most common forms of direct contact transmission given the extremely close and intimate contact that occurs during sex. Sexual transmission routes include vaginal or anal penetration that occurs when an object, such as a penis, finger or sex toy, is inserted into the vagina or anus during sexual intercourse. The lining of the vagina and anus is a mucous membrane. When penile penetration is involved, some pathogens can be transmitted from semen to the mucous membranes in the vaginal or anal canal. However, semen is not a prerequisite for infectious transmission, as pathogens can also be transmitted on the skin of the penis, fingers or other objects inserted into the vagina or anus. In addition to semen-facilitated transmission, inserting any object into the vagina or anus can cause minor to significant localized trauma. This can create opportunities for certain pathogens (for example, hepatitis B or C) to gain entry to the blood system, enhancing risk for blood-borne pathogen transmission.

Sexually transmitted infections can also occur through oral sexual transmission. Oral sexual transmission can occur when an individual has oral contact with any sexual organ (such as the penis or vulva and vagina). Like the vaginal or anal canals, the inner lining of the mouth is also a mucous membrane. This means that the mouth is susceptible to most sexual pathogens, including blood-borne pathogens. Although sexually transmitted infections are less likely to be transmitted via oral sex than vaginal or anal sex, there is still a risk (Saini et al., 2010).

It is important to note that penetrative sex does not necessarily have to occur for transmission to take place. The herpes virus, for example, is transmitted through contact with an area of skin that is shedding the virus, which may or may not have a visible lesion, and only skin-to-skin exposure to the virus is needed for transmission to occur. Therefore, barrier mechanisms, such as condoms, may not be effective in preventing herpes, as the virus shedding can occur around the sexual organs as well as on them.

Being infected with a sexually transmitted infection is an important risk factor for acquiring additional infections, including HIV and hepatitis B or C. This is because most sexually transmitted infections lead to the degradation of the skin or mucous membranes. Typically, this degraded tissue is the result of inflammation that occurs where the immune system is reacting to the presence of an infection, thus leading to skin sloughing, discharge and/or irritation. Wherever there is skin degradation in a mucous membrane, it increases risks for entry of other pathogens into the local tissue or the blood stream.

Activity 3.2

Read the case study below and then answer the questions that follow.

In January 2008, three people were diagnosed with acute hepatitis C virus (HCV). When it was discovered that the three individuals diagnosed with HCV had undergone endoscopy procedures at the same clinic, an epidemiological investigation was initiated. The investigation consisted of patient tracking and testing and a review of infection control practices at the clinic. The patient tracking and testing resulted in around 50,000 patients being contacted. From the 50,000 patients contacted, a further five in addition to the initial three were confirmed to be infected by HCV. Microbiological analysis revealed two distinct clusters of clinic-acquired HCV infections and a source patient related to each cluster. The review of infection control revealed single-use medication vials were used for multiple patients during anaesthesia administration and this likely resulted in patient-to-patient transmission of HCV due to contamination of the medication vials (Fischer *et al.*, 2010).

1. What are the specific infection control breaches observed in this scenario?
2. Based on your knowledge of routine practices, how should this clinic improve their infection control practices?
3. What systems-level issues should be considered by the government?

Feedback

1. Single-dose vials were used for multiple doses in more than one patient, which led to cross-contamination.

2. Staff should be properly trained in infection control. Syringes should not be reused when withdrawing medications for an individual patient or multiple patients. Single-use vials should never be used for multiple patients, and the use of multi-dose vials for multiple patients should be avoided. Monitoring systems need to be in place to ensure that single-use vials are not used for multiple patients.
3. Governments should put in place and enforce requirements that facilities maintain infection control using nationally recognized guidelines and that there is appropriate training for all staff. Governments have the power to regulate clinics and hospitals. This should require regular observations of procedures and formal assessments of infection control practices.

Contact transmission: indirect

Indirect contact transmission describes how a susceptible person becomes infected by contact with a surface or object that is contaminated with an infectious agent. Some infectious agents can survive on surfaces for an extended period of time. Inanimate (non-living) objects and surfaces which carry the infectious agent in indirect contact transmission are known as fomites. Common fomites include:

- Door knobs
- Household furniture
- Taps and other bathroom and toilet surfaces
- Cups, dishes, cutlery, trays
- Computer keyboards and telephones
- Pens, pencils, phones, office supplies
- Toys.

One type of indirect contact transmission is where faeces containing infectious agents contaminate a person's hands. Pathogens can then enter the bodies of individuals through food preparation or through contact with the contaminated hands. They then touch objects and surfaces such as cooking equipment that then infect other people. This is one type of faecal–oral transmission.

Contact transmission: droplet

Some infectious agents are expelled from the body in droplets of liquid. This occurs when people laugh, talk, spit, sneeze or cough. These droplets are small but not small enough to remain suspended in the air. They usually cannot travel more than about a metre from their point of origin. The droplets containing infectious agents enter the nose, eyes and mouth of potential hosts. In addition, the droplets can fall on to surrounding surfaces, enabling indirect contact transmission as described above. Examples of diseases that can be transmitted in this way include rhinovirus that causes the common cold, influenza, measles, diphtheria and bacterial meningitis.

Non-contact: airborne

Airborne transmission describes how tiny particles, which are made up partly or entirely of infectious agents, become suspended in the air. The particles can come from droplets expelled by infected people that have evaporated, leaving just the infectious agent. They can also come from infected dirt, urine or faecal matter, which has contaminated soil, bedding, clothing or flooring. Dust containing the infected particles then becomes dislodged when these are moved, cleaned or blown by wind. These particles are then breathed in by the potential host with the respiratory systems as the portal of entry. Because they are so small, the particles can penetrate into the upper and lower respiratory system. Unlike larger droplets described above, particles spread through airborne transmission can travel long distances on air currents. In order to be transmitted in this way, infectious agents must be able to remain alive for some time outside the body of a host. Given the small size of these particles, they are able to evade many barriers used to prevent infectious diseases, such as surgical masks. These factors make diseases that can be spread in this way very infectious. In addition, infectious diseases spread by airborne transmission can be very challenging to control, as this route of transmission does not require people to come into direct contact with one another. Examples of infectious diseases which can be spread in this way include measles, chickenpox and TB.

Non-contact: vector-borne

A vector is any living organism that transfers an infectious agent from one host to another. Frequently, the vector is insects. The vector carries the infectious agent from the reservoir to the new potential host. A biological vector carries the infectious agent in its own body, where it undergoes multiplication or development, and is essential to the life cycle of the infectious agent. A mechanical vector transports the infectious agent but is not essential to its life cycle, for example by carrying the infectious agent on its body. Often the portal of entry for the infectious agent is through the skin in the form of an insect bite. Infectious agents can also be spread through the faeces of a vector or on the outside of its body. For example, flies carry infectious agents on their feet and spread these by walking on food. One of the most common vectors is the mosquito, which transmits many diseases, including malaria, dengue and Rift Valley fever. However, it is important to bear in mind that vector-borne diseases are generally highly specific. This means that only a certain type of vector transmits a specific infectious agent. Table 3.2 gives details of some these vectors and the infectious diseases they transmit to humans.

Table 3.2 Vector-borne diseases and their vectors

Disease	Vector
Chikungunya	*Aedes* mosquito
Dengue fever	*Aedes* mosquito
Rift Valley fever	*Aedes* mosquito
Yellow fever	*Aedes* mosquito
Zika	*Aedes* mosquito
Malaria	*Anopheles* mosquito
Japanese encephalitis	*Culex* mosquito
Lymphatic filariasis	*Culex* mosquito
West Nile fever	*Culex* mosquito
Leishmaniasis	Sandfly
Sleeping sickness (African trypanosomiasis)	Tsetse flies
Onchocerciasis (river blindness)	Black flies
Schistosomiasis (bilharziasis)	Aquatic snails

Source: WHO (2016).

The physiology, habitat, quantity, range and behaviour of a vector will have a significant impact on how a vector-borne disease is transmitted. Therefore, it is important to identify and understand the particular vector responsible for transmitting a disease in order to develop effective control measures. For example, long-lasting bed nets treated with insecticide have not proved an effective preventative measure against visceral leishmaniasis whereas they have for malaria. This is probably because visceral leishmaniasis is transmitted through the bite of a sandfly. Sandflies are more likely to bite people when they are outside than mosquitoes, which transmit malaria, so any bed nets would have less impact on preventing sandfly–human contact than mosquito–human contact (Picado *et al.*, 2010).

Non-contact: vehicle-borne

A vehicle is an inanimate object or biological product that becomes contaminated with an infectious agent. The vehicle then comes into contact with a potential new host. It may be ingested or touched or penetrate the skin. It could also be introduced during medical treatment. Examples of common vehicles include cooking or eating utensils, clothing, toys, bedding, surgical or medical instruments (like catheters) or dressings. Water, food, drink and biological products like blood, serum, plasma, tissues or organs can act as vehicles.

In addition to indirect contact faecal–oral transmission, whereby faecal matter contaminates a person's hand, infectious agents can also be transmitted from faecal to oral using a vehicle. Food, water or cooking and eating utensils are usually the vehicle. Food and drinking water sources can become contaminated due to inadequate sanitation systems and infrastructure. Cooking and utensils washed in contaminated water can also act as the vehicle.

Another type of vehicle-borne transmission arises from intravenous drug use. The act of injecting drugs into a vein requires an individual to draw back on the syringe until they see blood in the chamber. This ensures that the needle is in the vein and that the drugs will not be injected into an interstitial space. Where a needle is shared with another user, the infectious agent from one person's blood can be transmitted to another person.

Other forms of vehicle-borne transmission can occur as a result of healthcare-bed related exposures, known as healthcare-associated infections (HCAIs). As the case study in Activity 3.2 showed, blood-borne pathogens can be introduced through inadequate infection control and improper use of equipment. Blood transfusions can also lead to the transmission of blood-borne pathogens, although the risks can be reduced substantially with the implementation of rigorous protocols to screen donors' blood.

Summary

This chapter has described the chain of infection and the role and types of reservoirs. It has also detailed the main portals of exit and entry, and the main modes of transmission, by which infectious agents leave existing hosts and enter new ones. These factors provide important information about how to control infectious disease by reducing or eliminating infectious agents, preventing them from spreading and reducing the susceptibility of potential new hosts to infection. Different infectious diseases require different types and combinations of control measures depending on how they are transmitted. The next section of this book goes on to discuss these control measures in more detail.

Further reading

Hutchinson, E. and Kovats, S. (2017) *Environment, Health and Sustainable Development*, 9th edn. London: Open University Press.

References

Centers for Disease Control and Prevention (CDC) (1992) *Principles of Epidemiology*, 2nd ed. Atlanta, GA: US Department of Health and Human Services.

Fischer, G.E., Schaefer, M.K., Labus, B.J., Sands, L., Rowley, P., Azzam, I.A. *et al*. (2010) Hepatitis C virus infections from unsafe injection practices at an endoscopy clinic in Las Vegas, Nevada, 2007–2008, *Clinical Infectious Diseases*, 51 (3): 267–273. Available at: https://doi.org/10.1086/653937

Hayden, D.T. (2002) Identifying reservoirs of infection: a conceptual and practical challenge, *Emerging Infectious Diseases*, 8 (12): 1468–1473.

Hutchinson, E. and Kovats, S. (2017) *Environment, Health and Sustainable Development*, 9th edn. London: Open University Press.

Jones, K.E., Patel, N.G., Levy, M.A., Storeygard, A., Balk, D., Gittleman J.L. *et al*. (2008) Global trends in emerging infectious diseases, *Nature*, 451 (7181): 990–993.

National Research Council (2009) 3. Drivers of zoonotic diseases, in G.T. Keusch, M. Pappaioanou, M.C. Gonzalez, K.A. Scott and P. Tsai, (eds.) *Sustaining Global Surveillance and Response to Emerging Zoonotic Diseases*, Committee on Achieving Sustainable Global Capacity for Surveillance and Response to Emerging Diseases of Zoonotic Origin. Washington, DC: National Academies Press. Available at: https://www.ncbi.nlm.nih.gov/books/NBK215318/ [accessed 12 January 2018].

One Health (2017) *One Health: a concept that became an approach and then a movement*. Available at: http://www.onehealthglobal.net/what-is-one-health/ [accessed 6 February 2017].

Picado, A., Singh, S.P., Rijal, S., Sundar, S., Ostyn, B., Chappuis, F. *et al*. (2010) Longlasting insecticidal nets for prevention of *Leishmania donovani* infection in India and Nepal: paired cluster randomised trial, *British Medical Journal*, 341: c6760.

Saini, R., Saini, S. and Sharma, S. (2010) Oral sex, oral health and orogenital infections, *Journal of Global Infectious Diseases*, 2 (1): 57–62.

Taylor, L.H., Latham, S.M. and Woolhouse, M.E. (2001) Risk factors for human disease emergence, *Philosophical Transactions of the Royal Society B: Biological Sciences*, 356 (1411): 983–989.

Webster, J.P., Borlase, A. and Rudge, J.W. (2017) Who acquires infection from whom and how? Disentangling multi-host and multi-mode transmission dynamics in the 'elimination' era, *Philosophical Transactions of the Royal Society B: Biological Sciences*, 372: 20160091.

World Health Organization (WHO) (2011) *Guidelines for the management of typhoid fever*. Available at: http://apps.who.int/medicinedocs/documents/s20994en/s20994en.pdf [accessed 7 February 2017].

World Health Organization (WHO) (2016) *Fact sheet on vector-borne diseases*. Available at: http://www.who.int/mediacentre/factsheets/fs387/en/ [accessed 7 February 2017].

Zinsstag, J., Schelling, E., Waltner-Toews, D. and Tanner, M. (2011) From 'one medicine' to 'one health' and systemic approaches to health and well-being, *Preventive Veterinary Medicine*, 101 (3/4): 148–156.

SECTION 2

Measures to control communicable disease

Surveillance

Liza Cragg and James Rudge

4

Overview

Section 1 of this book introduced key concepts in the control of communicable disease, including a brief history of how control developed and an explanation of the causes and transmission of communicable disease. Section 2 now turns to the measures that are used to control communicable disease. This chapter explains the crucial role surveillance plays in controlling communicable diseases, exploring what surveillance is and what it is used for. It describes the overall design of a surveillance system and explains the activities that make up communicable disease surveillance, including the types of data that are used, how they are collected and analysed, and what they can be used for. Finally, the chapter describes the essential features of a communicable diseases surveillance system.

Learning objectives

After reading this chapter, you will be able to:

• explain the role that surveillance plays in communicable disease control
• describe the activities involved in communicable disease surveillance
• explain the types of data that are used in communicable disease surveillance and different approaches to collecting data
• describe the key features of a communicable disease surveillance system

Key terms

Active surveillance: Surveillance that includes actively contacting health providers and laboratories to report cases of disease, which can include active case finding. Requires reporting of negative cases.

Enhanced surveillance: Collection of more detailed data than would ordinarily be collected in passive surveillance.

Notifiable disease: Any disease that is required by law to be reported to government authorities.

Passive surveillance: Where health facilities routinely record and report data from patients on defined events to the relevant health authorities.

Reporting unit: A health facility or laboratory that submits data to a surveillance system.

Sentinel surveillance: A type of sample surveillance, with reporting units situated at selected sites within a given area.

Surveillance: The continuous, systematic collection, analysis and interpretation of health-related data needed for the planning, implementation and evaluation of public health practice.

Syndromic surveillance: The process of collecting surveillance data on the presence of specific symptoms, rather than data on cases with confirmed diagnoses.

What is surveillance and what is it for?

The World Health Organization (WHO) defines public health surveillance as 'the continuous, systematic collection, analysis and interpretation of health-related data needed for the planning, implementation, and evaluation of public health practice' (WHO, 2016). The overall objective of public health surveillance is to provide accurate information in a timely way to enable appropriate public health action. Surveillance for specific public health issues requires objectives and methods tailored to that issue. For example, a surveillance system for non-communicable diseases will require different data that will be used for different purposes than one for infectious diseases (Nsubuga et al., 2006). Ensuring an effective surveillance system is in place and functioning well can be essential for the control of communicable disease for reasons that are explained in this chapter.

The overall design of a surveillance system

Surveillance systems will be designed according to the health issues they explore. However, some activities remain constant whatever public health issue the surveillance system is concerned with. These activities form a cycle, as shown in Figure 4.1.

The first step is to define the specific objectives of the surveillance system so the relevant data can be collected. This includes specifying the population that is under surveillance and what the surveillance system is seeking to identify. The specific objectives of a surveillance system for communicable disease are outlined in the next section of this chapter. The sources of the data and the methods for collecting it need also to be specified. The data itself then needs to be generated and collected. Next, the data should be analysed. The different types of data that are often used in surveillance systems for communicable disease and methods for analysing these data are described later in this chapter. The analysed data and relevant conclusions need to be presented clearly and communicated to those responsible for making decisions and taking action. Surveillance data should also be used to evaluate the effectiveness of the action taken. This evaluation may generate new areas of concern that require further surveillance, or indeed indicate that previous threats have reduced, which means the surveillance system data requirements and methods may need to be revised accordingly. Throughout this process, it is important to bear in mind that recording and collecting data requires time and effort that can only be justified if it is analysed and used. Collecting data that is not analysed and used is a waste of resources.

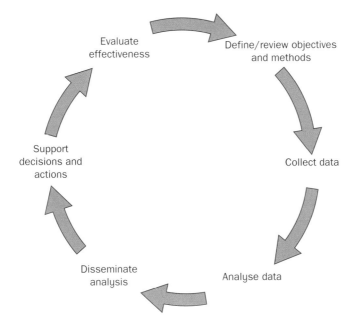

Figure 4.1 The overall design of a surveillance system

Components of a communicable disease surveillance system

Objectives

The specific objectives of communicable disease surveillance include:

• providing an early warning system to detect outbreaks;
• identifying communicable disease cases and their importance;

- monitoring communicable disease trends;
- detecting changes in infectious agents, including development of antibiotic resistance;
- evaluating the effectiveness of communicable disease control and prevention measures;
- providing an evidence base for formulation of policy, regulations and guidelines;
- providing data and information for research.

Most countries have national communicable disease surveillance systems in operation that seek to identify cases of specific diseases, particularly vaccine-preventable, highly infectious or potentially serious diseases. These typically look at the entire population. Many countries also collect additional data to look at certain populations in more detail. These might include high-risk groups, such as older people or pregnant women, or particular geographical areas that are more prone to outbreaks. Most countries also have legislation that specifies notifiable diseases. A notifiable disease is any disease that is required by law to be reported to government authorities so that they can ensure public health investigation or follow-up to reduce the risk of further spread. National-level surveillance systems feed into global surveillance overseen by the WHO and other United Nations (UN) agencies (WHO, 2017). The International Health Regulations (IHRs) are legally binding requirements for countries to help prevent and respond to acute public health risks that have the potential to cross borders and threaten people worldwide. The IHRs require countries to report certain disease outbreaks to the WHO. This requirement includes developing and maintaining core capacities for communicable disease surveillance and response (WHO, 2005). The IHRs played a key role in the global response to the recent pandemic caused by the influenza A(H1N1)pdm09 strain, first detected in North America in 2009 (Fineberg, 2014).

Data collection

Five main approaches exist to generate and collect data in communicable disease surveillance systems: passive surveillance, active surveillance, enhanced surveillance, sentinel surveillance and syndromic surveillance. These may be used individually or in combination, depending on the epidemiological, clinical and biological characteristics of the communicable disease, and the resources and data that are available in the prevailing circumstances. It is worth noting that precise definitions for these different types of surveillance can vary between contexts and sources, but the key features and examples of each approach are described in turn next.

Passive surveillance

Health systems include mechanisms for health facilities to routinely record and report data from patients on defined events, such as confirmed or suspected cases of specific diseases. This is known as passive surveillance and is the most commonly used form of disease surveillance. There is no active search for cases of disease. Instead, every healthcare provider, including primary care practices, hospitals, laboratories, community nurses and private practices, reports cases of diseases and other conditions to a higher administrative level. Each healthcare provider submitting data is known as a reporting unit. In most countries, every healthcare provider is required to submit a monthly report in a standard format. Sometimes this may be more frequently, depending on the context and specific disease. Data is then aggregated and analysed at the local, regional and national levels to provide information on defined events.

Passive surveillance has several advantages. It is cost-effective because it relies on existing systems and it generally covers wide geographical areas (usually a whole country), thereby enabling the monitoring of trends over time and place. However, it also has some disadvantages. It can only capture a minimum amount of information, such as numbers of cases testing positive for a specified disease and basic demographic information. It relies on healthcare providers having the capacity to diagnose accurately the diseases it covers. In some countries or areas, the required diagnostic facilities may not be available. In addition, healthcare workers may lack the motivation or ability to complete the surveillance in a timely way. While in some countries the requirements for passive surveillance may be strictly enforced, with penalties for healthcare providers who fail to provide the necessary data, in others reporting requirements may not be enforced. This means data may not be complete, which affects the reliability of surveillance. In addition, passive surveillance does not require negative reporting, meaning that if a reporting unit has no cases, it does not have to compile a report. Passive surveillance also requires patients to seek health care in order for cases to be identified. In contexts where accessing health care is difficult due to cost, distance or other constraints, passive surveillance may not be effective. Also, people may be reluctant to seek care for conditions where there is fear of stigma, such as sexually transmitted infections, so passive surveillance may not adequately capture these conditions. Actions to improve passive surveillance include training for healthcare providers, ensuring reporting is made as simple as possible, providing feedback on reporting and prompt follow-up of missed reporting.

Active surveillance

Active surveillance involves the health department or authority responsible for communicable disease surveillance contacting healthcare providers to identify cases and collect data in relation to them. This may include action

Box 4.1:   Example of a surveillance form for measles, mumps and rubella used in England

Surveillance form for confirmed measles/mumps/rubella cases

Name of case: _____ DOB: _____ Sex: M/F

Date of onset of illness: _____ Date of sample: _____

Epidemiological features

1. Vaccination history and dates:

Vaccine	Given?		Make & batch no	Date given (if known)
MMR	yes ☐	no ☐		_____
MMR2	yes ☐	no ☐		_____
Measles	yes ☐	no ☐		_____
MR	yes ☐	no ☐		_____
Rubella	yes ☐	no ☐		_____

2. Was the patient pregnant?   Yes ☐   No ☐

   If yes, what was the gestational age at time of test? . . . .

   Is the woman planning to continue with her pregnancy?   Yes ☐   No ☐

   If yes: what is her EDD? _____

   Where is she planning to deliver? _____

   Who is her obstetrician? _____

3. Was the patient hospitalised?   Yes ☐   No ☐

   If yes, please state with what condition and list any complications/outcome:

   _____

   _____

4. History of foreign travel in the month before onset?   Yes ☐   No ☐

   If yes, to where: _____Date of return: _____

5. Contact with a similar illness in the month before onset?   Yes ☐   No ☐

   If yes: Name of case (if known): _____

             Area/country of residence: _____

             If at school, please state school name: _____

   Was the illness in the contact investigated?   Yes ☐   No ☐   not sure ☐

   If yes, to which laboratory were the tests sent? _____

6. Any other details: _____

   _____

7. Requesting doctor name: _____

   GP name and address: _____

   _____

Patient postcode: _____ Completed by: _____

Thank you for your help. Please return to:
Public Health England, CIDSC, Immunisation Department,

Source: Public Health England.

to follow up patients and confirm diagnoses through questionnaires, examinations and/or diagnostic tests. It may include active case finding, whereby healthcare providers screen individuals or population groups for diseases. For example, active case finding is used for tuberculosis surveillance in high-risk populations in some countries. It may also include contact tracing, which means identifying and contacting people that patients may have had contact with to determine whether they have become infected. In addition, active surveillance requires negative reporting, meaning that if a reporting unit has no cases they are required to send in a report specifying this. Active surveillance is extremely resource-intensive. Therefore, it is used when it is important that surveillance information is complete, such as for diseases that have the potential to cause significant morbidity and mortality (for example, meningococcal infection, viral haemorrhagic fever, tuberculosis (TB), rabies and diphtheria) and rare diseases (for example, Reye syndrome, a rare but serious condition affecting children). One such unit is the British Paediatric Surveillance Unit (BPSU), which undertakes active surveillance of rare diseases and infections in children (Lynn *et al.*, 2016). Active surveillance is often used as a short-term measure during a period of elevated risk, for example during the season when outbreaks of influenza are more likely.

Enhanced surveillance

Precise definitions for enhanced surveillance can vary, but in general the term refers to the collection of a more comprehensive dataset than would normally be collected through passive surveillance. Because enhanced surveillance involves active efforts to collect the additional data, it is sometimes considered a special form of active surveillance. Enhanced surveillance can involve following up events reported through passive surveillance to obtain additional data. This additional information may include possible exposures and more detailed clinical information. The information will normally be collected by contacting the health facility responsible for reporting the diagnosis and asking for additional details, or by contacting the patient directly. Enhanced surveillance tends to be used where it becomes clear that the provisions of the passive surveillance system are not sufficient for an adequate response to an emerging outbreak. For example, in 2011 there was an outbreak of bloody diarrhoea and haemolytic uraemic syndrome (HUS) caused by Shiga toxin/verotoxin-producing *Escherichia coli* in Germany. An enhanced surveillance system was put in place that supplemented the existing passive surveillance with the following:

- centralizing the epidemiological information exchange;
- accelerating the data flow to the national level;
- implementing a syndromic surveillance system for bloody diarrhoea in emergency departments;
- assessing the capacities for hemolytic uremic syndrome (HUS) in Germany;
- initiating active laboratory surveillance (Wadl *et al.*, 2011).

Sentinel surveillance

Sentinel surveillance involves a selection of reporting units (sentinel sites) collecting data from a sample of the population rather than the entire population. Sentinel surveillance is used when high-quality data are needed that cannot be obtained through the passive surveillance system. Instead of all health facilities acting as reporting units, a number of facilities of the type that have a high probability of seeing cases of the disease under surveillance are selected, for example general practitioners (GPs) for influenza. The network of facilities involved in a sentinel surveillance system will typically also include laboratories that can correctly identify and characterize precise infectious agents. In England, for example, influenza surveillance relies partly on a sentinel surveillance network of approximately 100 GPs who report the number of weekly consultations for influenza-like illness (ILI). Around 85 of these sites also obtain nose and throat swabs from ILI patients, which are sent to the Virus Reference Department of Public Health England for virus isolation and characterization. This provides timely information on the incidence of ILI, the proportion of patients with ILI that are positive for influenza, and the influenza strains in circulation. These data are also provided to the WHO, thus feeding into a global surveillance system to guide in the annual formulation of the influenza vaccine (Public Health England, 2014).

Sentinel surveillance can provide high-quality data in a timely and cost-effective manner. It is most commonly used for monitoring trends in diseases that are common and widespread such as varicella, gastroenteritis and common acute respiratory viruses. It has also been used effectively in low-income countries to improve surveillance of particular diseases during and after outbreak responses (Randrianasolo *et al.*, 2010). However, it has a number of limitations. Because it only covers a small proportion of the population, it is not useful to detect rare diseases. It also does not identify cases outside the catchment areas of the selected reporting units. Additionally, sentinel reporting units need to be carefully selected so as to be representative of the population of interest or it can lead to erroneous conclusions about trends. Patients must also be able to access the health facilities that act as reporting units. Finally, this type of surveillance requires that healthcare providers have the necessary capacity and willingness to participate.

Syndromic surveillance

Syndromic surveillance involves continuous and systematic collection of data on the presence of specific symptoms, rather than data on cases with confirmed diagnoses. It relies on data collected at sources such as accident and emergency hospital units, GP surgeries, out-of-hours services and health advice lines. It is used to detect potential threats at an early stage. Syndromic surveillance is sometimes used at mass gathering events, where lots of people from different parts of the world come together in the same place when there is the potential for an infectious agent to be introduced and for an outbreak to spread rapidly. It can also be used to monitor seasonal trends, for example influenza-like illness as a proxy for influenza virus.

This type of surveillance data has a number of advantages. It can be generated very quickly, often within 12 hours of initiation. Therefore, it is useful to rapidly conduct surveillance for new and emerging issues. It can be effective in additional case finding when an outbreak has already been identified and confirmed. It is also useful for alleviating concerns among communities about the need for action to identify potential cases when outbreaks are occurring elsewhere. However, syndromic surveillance also has significant limitations. It is very sensitive but has low specificity and so can lead to false alarms. The fact that many symptoms are not disease-specific potentially limits the disease outbreaks that can be detected. The incubation period of the infectious agents may also affect the utility of this approach, as patients may not develop symptoms until sometime after they become infected (Hope *et al.*, 2006).

✎ Activity 4.1

Imagine you are required to develop a syndromic surveillance pro-gramme for a mass gathering event such as an Olympic Games.

1. Develop aims for the syndromic surveillance programme.
2. Where would you collect data from or, in other words, what would be the reporting units?
3. How often would you collect and analyse the data and why?
4. What would you be looking for when analysing the data?

Feedback

In preparation for the London 2012 Olympics, the UK public health authority, the Health Protection Agency, introduced a syndromic surveil-lance system. The feedback below comes from the final surveillance report produced (Health Protection Agency, 2013).

1. The aims of a syndromic surveillance programme for a mass gathering event would include:
   • To provide early warning of incidents
   • To describe the extent and spread of known incidents ('situational awareness')
   • To provide reassurance about the lack of impact of incidents.
2. Data should be collected from reporting units including all healthcare providers accessible to people in the area of the event, any national

health telephone advice line, primary care practices, out-of-hours primary care providers and hospital emergency departments.

3. Analysis of mass gathering event data should be undertaken at least once every 24 hours to ensure that any potential incidents are identified immediately.

4. When analysing the data, you should be looking for any increases in reported symptoms that might indicate the beginning of an outbreak. In order to identify these, it is important to calculate baselines that show normal levels of symptoms. These may need to take into account potential confounding factors, including seasonal effects, days of the week, holidays and changes in coverage. Significant increases above these baselines should generate 'alarms' that need to be investigated further.

Analysis

Analysis of surveillance data for communicable disease control uses quantitative assessment to explore the *pattern* of specific diseases according to:

• *Person*: who is being affected and who is at risk?
• *Time*: how does it compare to last year/month/week and when did this start?
• *Place*: where is it happening?

Person analysis looks at the attributes of the patients, including their age group, sex and ethnicity with a view to identifying if any one group is affected more than another and, if so, to investigate why. It is also important to highlight if any vulnerable groups are affected. For example, cases of rubella among women of childbearing age are potentially serious because of the risk of congenital rubella syndrome (CRS).

Time analysis looks at how cases of disease are distributed over different time periods. This may mean comparing the number of cases with those at the same point in previous years to see if the current year represents a change. Analysis can include looking at new cases at monthly or weekly intervals to identify seasonal trends or outbreaks. It could even include analysis on a daily basis for significant outbreaks or events where it is essential to identify potential trends immediately. The date used for analysis may be defined as the date of symptom onset or the date of diagnosis. Numbers analysed may be new cases in a defined time period or cumulative cases. Distribution of cases over time is usually presented as a graph with time on the x-axis and number of cases on the y-axis. Figure 4.2 provides an example.

Place analysis seeks to identify patterns of disease according to geographical location. It compares the number of new cases in different

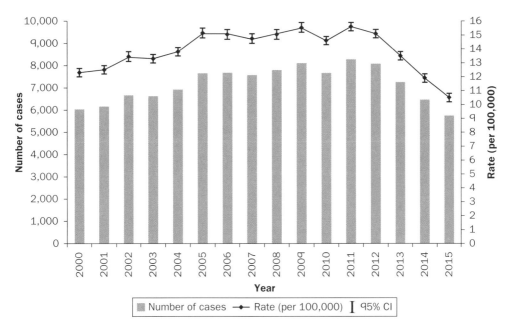

Figure 4.2 Tuberculosis (TB) case notifications and rates, England, 2000–2015

Source: Public Health England (2016).

geographical units. The unit used for comparison may be very small, such as a specific institution (for example, a school or workplace) or neighbourhood, or larger such as city, region or even country. Geographical maps are frequently used to display the analysis of data according to place. An example of mapping is given in Figure 4.3.

In addition to exploring patterns of disease, analysis also needs to identify the *frequency* of the disease(s) under surveillance. This entails comparing the number of cases with a given denominator. The denominator used will often be the size of the population, although this is not always possible or appropriate, such as when the catchment area is unknown. In this case, other denominators, such as the total number of patients presenting at the reporting units within a given period, may be chosen.

Analysis of surveillance data should also aim to identify any factors that may impact on the accuracy of findings. This could include incomplete or incorrect data recording and delays in reporting. For example, if one reporting unit has failed to submit their monthly data, this will impact on the total number of cases for that month for comparison with other time periods and places. The potential importance of these factors should be assessed and, if possible, adjusted for in the analysis, with any resulting limitations clearly acknowledged.

Analysis of surveillance data involves the application of core epidemiological concepts and tools. These are explained in more detail in *Introduction*

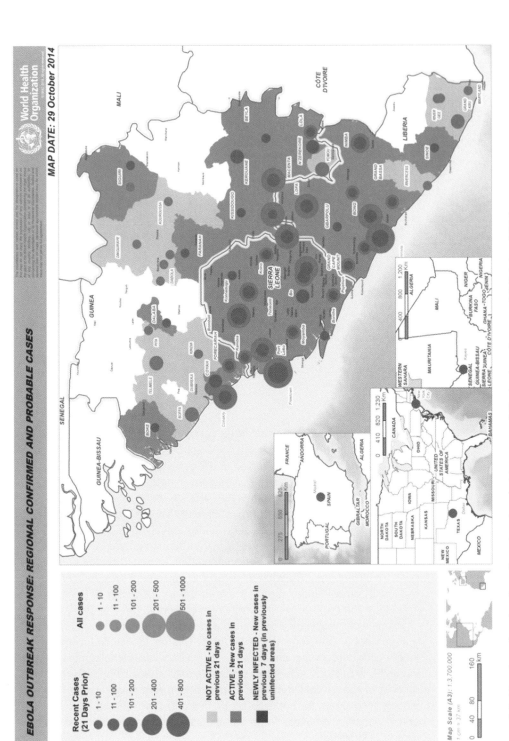

Figure 4.3 Mapping of regional confirmed and probable cases of Ebola virus disease, 29 October 2014

Source: WHO (2014).

to Epidemiology (Carneiro and Howard, 2011), which is part of the Understanding Public Health series. They include:

- *Prevalence*: the total number of individuals alive in a population who have a specific disease or other condition, either during a period of time (period prevalence) or at a particular point in time (point prevalence), usually expressed as a percentage of the population.
- *Incidence*: the number of individuals who develop a specific disease or other condition during a particular time period (such as a month or year), usually reported in relation to the size of the population at risk of developing the disease (for example, per 100,000 people per year).
- *Epidemic curve* (epi curve): shows the number of cases (for example, by date of illness onset or date of diagnosis) in an outbreak over time.
- *Case fatality rate*: the proportion of cases of a specified disease or condition which are fatal within a specified time.
- *Overall attack rate*: the total number of new cases divided by the total population for a given outbreak or time period.
- *Primary case*: the person who first brings a disease into a group of people.
- *Secondary cases*: the people infected by the primary case.
- *Index case*: the first case to come to the attention of the health authorities.
- *Epidemic*: the occurrence of more cases of a disease than expected in a given area or among a specific group of persons during a given time period.
- *Endemic*: the constant presence of an infectious agent or disease within a given geographic area or population.
- *Pandemic*: an epidemic that spreads to several continents.

Dissemination

It is important to disseminate the analysis of surveillance data so it can be used to inform decision-making on the control of communicable disease. Dissemination involves presenting the analysis in a format appropriate for the target audience. This requires identifying the target audience in advance and understanding their information needs and priorities. Audiences may include decision-makers, programme planners, clinicians, researchers, the public and patients. Each of these audiences will be using the information to make different types of decisions and will have different levels of expertise. The level of detail and technical complexity of the information will need to be tailored to their needs. The information will also need to be presented in different formats, including newsletters, policy briefings, presentations and posters.

Surveillance data should generally be available to the public. Datasets and reports describing which data are available for each key population by geographical area should be available. The methodology for collecting and analysing the data and any potential limitations should also be explained. This can be done through the relevant health authority website.

Informing decision-making and action

The overall objective of a communicable disease surveillance system is to enable informed decision-making and effective action. There are many different types of decisions and actions that surveillance data can be used to inform. Activity 4.2 explores some of these. Exploring whether a surveillance system has been used to inform action in practice, and identifying which action and by whom is a good way of testing its overall usefulness.

 Activity 4.2

Think of examples of communicable disease surveillance information materials. Who do you think they are aimed at? What type of decisions and action do you think they are seeking to inform?

Feedback

Examples of information materials for communicable disease surveillance and their intended audiences include:

• Regular newsletters produced by national health authorities analysing surveillance data aimed at policy-makers, healthcare providers, non-governmental organizations (NGOs) and scientists. For examples, see the journal *Communicable Diseases Intelligence* produced by the Department of Health of the Australian Government (available at: http://www.health.gov.au/internet/main/publishing.nsf/Content/cdi4004-1) and the *Morbidity and Mortality Weekly Report* (MMWR) series prepared by the Centers for Disease Control and Prevention (CDC) in the USA (available at: https://www.cdc.gov/mmwr/index2016.html).
• Weekly updates of cases of notifiable diseases, aimed at policy-makers, health providers and scientists. See, for example, analysis of data for statutory notifications of infectious diseases (NOIDS) in England and Wales in 2016 (available at: https://www.gov.uk/government/publications/notifiable-diseases-weekly-report-2016).
• Global surveillance reports prepared by the WHO on outbreaks aimed at policy-makers, healthcare providers, NGOs and scientists. These are available on the WHO website (http://www.who.int/emergencies).
• Mass media campaigns using newspapers, television, radio and other media to tell people about the arrival of the influenza season and the need for vaccination aimed at patients and the public.
• Annual reports for specific diseases aimed at policy-makers, health providers and scientists. See, for example, *Tuberculosis in England 2016 Report* (Public Health England, 2016)

Examples of types of decisions and actions that surveillance data could be used to inform include: policy-makers allocating resources to diseases that are becoming more significant; healthcare providers increasing prevention measures for hospital-acquired infections; members of the public deciding whether to have influenza vaccinations; public health authorities launching new information campaigns to encourage parents to have their children vaccinated; scientists undertaking research into infectious agents showing drug resistance; local food standards agency action against a restaurant suspected of causing food poisoning; an NGO advocating for more resources for a particular population group or geographical area identified to be at high risk of a particular disease.

Evaluate the effectiveness of action

Communicable disease surveillance data also needs to be used to evaluate the effectiveness of the action taken. If surveillance data shows that the action taken is not having the intended epidemiological impact, this suggests that intervention strategies need to be revised. It may also indicate that the surveillance system itself needs to be modified. For example, data may need to be collected more frequently, or more rigorously in specific population groups or geographical areas. Conversely, if surveillance data suggests an outbreak is over, it may be appropriate to reduce surveillance after a sufficient interval.

Requirements of a communicable disease surveillance system

In order to meet the objectives described earlier in this chapter, a communicable disease surveillance system must fulfil several requirements. It must be (WHO, 2006):

- *Systematic*: Communicable disease surveillance must be systematic, which means there should be clearly defined processes for collecting information that are applied in the same way in different locations. It also requires that there are systems in place to verify that all reporting sites included in the system provide the data needed.
- *Sensitive*: Surveillance must be sensitive enough to capture a sufficient number of events or conditions of interest. For example, it must be able to capture new cases of an infectious disease in order to identify the beginning of an outbreak. Sensitivity in surveillance refers to the proportion of actual cases in a population that are detected and notified through the system. High sensitivity is essential for rare or potentially serious events that could signal an outbreak, such as a new case of measles. Lower sensitivity is likely to be acceptable for

more common and less threatening events, for example cases of rhinovirus. It is crucial the level of sensitivity is consistent, or at least measured or acknowledged in some way, as changes in sensitivity could lead to false conclusions regarding temporal patterns in the number of true cases.

- *Specific*: Surveillance must be able to identify particular pathogens or events that are significant, thus allowing differentiation from other pathogens or events. Inadequate specificity could lead to inflated estimates of disease prevalence and incidence. It could also overwhelm surveillance systems involved in outbreak detection by triggering too many 'false alarms' that require further investigation.

- *Timely*: The most important measure of timeliness is whether data is submitted, analysed and disseminated in time to ensure that appropriate actions can be planned and implemented as soon as possible based on the most recent evidence. Timeliness of surveillance data is particularly important for outbreak detection so that immediate action can be taken to identify and control the source(s) and thus minimize further spread. Specific measures of timeliness include the time between the occurrence of an event and its subsequent identification; the time between identification and notification to the relevant authorities; and the timeliness of routine (for example, weekly and monthly) report submissions.

- *Useful*: As explained above, communicable disease surveillance has several objectives. The usefulness of a surveillance system depends on its ability to achieve these objectives.

- *Representative*: The surveillance system must accurately portray the incidence of a health event in a population. In order to generalize about a community from surveillance data, the system must be representative. This means that information should generally be collected from geographical areas, healthcare providers and population groups in accordance with their respective size and importance. One of the main challenges for surveillance of communicable disease in contexts where the private sector provides a significant proportion of health care is ensuring private sector providers are incorporated in surveillance. For example, recent research in India identified very significant under-reporting of TB because many patients are seen in the private healthcare sector, which is not integrated into the country's disease surveillance programme (Arinaminpathy *et al.*, 2016).

- *Acceptable*: The surveillance system must be acceptable to staff or they are unlikely to implement it. It must also be acceptable to patients whose data will be stored on the systems. Public health surveillance, including communicable disease surveillance, does not generally require explicit patient consent. However, it is important that the surveillance system is well-designed, engages affected communities, collects the minimum data necessary, stores data securely and uses data for public health action (Lee *et al.*, 2012). Most countries have data protection legislation and ethical standards that must be observed. In countries where data protection legislation and ethical standards are not in place, good practice guidance should be used.

- *User-friendly*: The surveillance system must not be so complex or time-consuming that it is very difficult for the staff responsible to implement it correctly and accurately. It is important that the system is developed with attention to institutional and human resource capacity, including the educational and professional level of the staff that will be responsible for implementing it. Training in how to use the system should also be provided on a regular basis.

 Activity 4.3

Read the following scenario and consider the questions that follow.

Matthew is a 21-year-old university student, who identifies as being bisexual. He is currently sexually active with several different partners. Matthew went to a walk-in clinic for his annual human immunodeficiency virus (HIV) screening test. During his visit he was questioned about risk factors and counselled to have additional tests done for sexually transmitted infections (STIs). Several days later Matthew received a telephone call from the clinic advising him that he had tested positive for syphilis, which is a notifiable disease, and asking him to return there for treatment. During his return visit to the clinic, a nurse met with him and discussed notifying his previous sexual partners. The nurse offered Matthew support to do it himself, and also offered for the clinic to contact his partners by letter or phone and advise them to go for a check-up. The nurse explained that all his details would remain totally confidential.

1. Between Matthew having had the blood test and receiving the telephone call from the clinic, describe what type of surveillance you think has occurred and why?
2. When the nurse meets Matthew on his return visit to the clinic and discusses his sexual history, what type of surveillance is this an example of and why?
3. Why is the type of surveillance identified in question 2 appropriate/ important for STI surveillance?

Feedback

1. Behind the scenes, the clinician and laboratory will have reported the results of the positive syphilis test to the public health authority, as it is identified as a notifiable disease. This is an example of passive

surveillance, as the system relies on health facilities routinely reporting defined events (in this instance, the case of a notifiable disease) to a health authority.

2. This is an example of enhanced surveillance, as the nurse is actively following up on information on a confirmed case to obtain more comprehensive data than would normally be collected through passive surveillance.

3. Many STIs have no immediate symptoms, so people can be infected without realizing it. One of the main mechanisms available to prevent and control spread and complications associated with STIs is to identify, test and treat people who have potentially been exposed. In the case of Matthew and his sexual partners, they are all potentially at risk for contracting syphilis and developing complications. This surveillance improves the health outcomes of the individuals affected by identifying them and treating them. Treating affected individuals can also reduce transmission to others. Conducting this type of surveillance on STIs can provide important information on the incidence and prevalence of infections, as well as information on behavioural risk factors, within high-risk populations. It can indicate if there is a need to improve information and/or services or to target services at specific communities who have higher than average incidence. While passive surveillance would provide some information on incidence, it would not enable partners to be contacted and treated. Active surveillance would require more resources, which would generally not be warranted for the disease concerned unless there was evidence of an unexplained increase in cases.

Summary

Surveillance is the cornerstone of communicable disease control. It is through surveillance that outbreaks can be identified early so that appropriate measures to prevent them spreading can be put in place. Surveillance is also essential to monitor trends in diseases and to evaluate the effectiveness of ongoing control activities, such as vaccination. Surveillance involves a number of interdependent activities, including defining objectives and methods; collecting, analysing and interpreting data; disseminating information; informing decisions; and evaluating the effectiveness of action. Different approaches to collecting surveillance data include passive surveillance, active surveillance, enhanced surveillance, syndromic surveillance and sentinel surveillance. An important indicator of the effectiveness of a surveillance system is whether it is used to inform decision-making. For a communicable disease surveillance system to be effective, it must be systematic, sensitive, specific, timely, representative, acceptable and user-friendly.

Further reading

Last, J.M. (2008) *A Dictionary of Epidemiology*. Oxford: Oxford University Press.

References

Arinaminpathy, N., Batra, D., Khaparde, S., Vualnam, T., Maheshwari, N., Sharma, L. *et al.* (2016) The number of privately treated tuberculosis cases in India: an estimation from drug sales data, *The Lancet Infectious Diseases*, 16 (11): 1255–1260.

Carneiro, I. and Howard, N. (2011) *Introduction to Epidemiology*. Maidenhead: Open University Press.

Fineberg, H. (2014) Pandemic preparedness and response – lessons from the H1N1 influenza of 2009, *New England Journal of Medicine*, 370: 1335–1342.

Health Protection Agency (2013) *Syndromic Surveillance Report: London 2012 Olympic and Paralympic Games*. Available at: https://www.gov.uk/government/uploads/system/uploads/attachment_data/file/398954/2.6__Syndromic_Surveillance_London_2012_report.pdf [accessed 14 February 2017].

Hope, K., Durrheim, D.N., d'Espaignet, E.T. and Dalton, C. (2006) Syndromic surveillance: is it a useful tool for local outbreak detection?, *Journal of Epidemiology and Community Health*, 60 (5): 374–375.

Lee, L.M., Heilig, C.M. and White, A. (2012) Ethical justification for conducting public health surveillance without patient consent, *American Journal of Public Health*, 102 (1): 38–44.

Lynn, R.M., Avis, J.L. and Reading, R. (eds.) (2016) *British Paediatric Surveillance Unit 30th Anniversary Report: Facilitating childhood rare disease research for over 30 years*. London: British Paediatric Surveillance Unit. Available at: www.rcpch.ac.uk/bpsu/30yearreport [accessed 15 May 2017].

Nsubuga, P., White, M.E., Thacker, S.B., Anderson, M.A., Blount, S.B., Broome, C.V. *et al.* (2006) Public health surveillance: a tool for targeting and monitoring interventions, in D.T. Jamison, J.G. Breman, A.R. Measham, G. Alleyne, M. Claeson, D.B. Evans *et al.* (eds.) *Disease Control Priorities in Developing Countries*, 2nd edn. Washington, DC: The World Bank/New York: Oxford University Press. Available at: https://www.ncbi.nlm.nih.gov/books/NBK11770/.

Public Health England (2014) *Sources of UK flu data: influenza surveillance in the UK*. Available at: https://www.gov.uk/guidance/sources-of-uk-flu-data-influenza-surveillance-in-the-uk [accessed 14 September 2017].

Public Health England (2016) *Tuberculosis in England: 2016 report*. London: Tuberculosis Section, Centre for Infectious Disease Surveillance and Control, National Infection Service. PHE. Available at: https://www.tbalert.org/wp-content/uploads/2016/09/PHE_TB_Annual_Report_2016.pdf [accessed 14 February 2017].

Randrianasolo, L., Raoelina, Y., Ratsitorahina, M., Ravolomanana, L., Andriamandimby, S., Heraud, J.-M. *et al.* (2010) Sentinel surveillance system for early outbreak detection in Madagascar, *BMC Public Health*, 10 (1): 31.

Wadl, M., Rieck, T., Nachtnebel, M., Greutélaers, B., van der Heiden, M., Altmann, D. *et al.* (2011) Enhanced surveillance during a large outbreak of bloody diarrhoea and haemolytic uraemic syndrome caused by Shiga toxin/verotoxin-producing *Escherichia coli* in Germany, May to June 2011, *Eurosurveillance*, 16 (24): pii=19893.

World Health Organization (WHO) (2005) *International Health Regulations (IHR)*, 3rd edn. Geneva: WHO. Available at: http://www.who.int/ihr/publications/9789241580496/en/ [accessed 9 February 2017].

World Health Organization (WHO) (2006) *Communicable disease surveillance and response systems: Guide to monitoring and evaluating*. Geneva: WHO. Available at: http://www.who.int/csr/resources/publications/surveillance/WHO_CDS_EPR_LYO_2006_2.pdf [accessed 9 February 2017].

World Health Organization (WHO) (2014) *Ebola outbreak response: Regional confirmed and probable cases*, Map date 29 October 2014. Geneva: WHO. Available at: http://www.who.int/csr/disease/ebola/photos/geographic-map-29-oct-2014.png?ua=1.

World Health Organization (WHO) (2016) *Public health surveillance factsheet*. Geneva: WHO. Available at: http://www.who.int/topics/public_health_surveillance/en/ [accessed 9 February 2017].

World Health Organization (WHO) (2017) *Fact sheet on immunization surveillance, assessment and monitoring*. Geneva: WHO. Available at: http://www.who.int/immunization/monitoring_surveillance/en/ [accessed 9 February 2017].

Vaccination

Liza Cragg and James Rudge

Overview

The previous chapter looked at the crucial role surveillance plays in identifying outbreaks, monitoring trends, designing measures to control communicable disease and evaluating their effectiveness. This chapter explains
how vaccination is used to prevent and control communicable disease. It
starts by briefly describing the history of vaccination and the Expanded
Programme of Immunization. It goes on to explain how vaccination works
and the types of vaccine that are currently available. It then describes the
main strategies used to design and deliver vaccination programmes, before
going on to explore practical considerations for their success and concepts
in monitoring vaccination programmes. Finally, it provides an overview of
some of the challenges involved.

Learning objectives

After reading this chapter, you will be able to:

- understand the main types of vaccine available
- describe the key features of the Expanded Programme of Immunization
- define herd immunity and the basic reproduction number, R_0, and explain
  why these concepts are important for vaccination programmes
- understand different strategies used to implement vaccination and
  when they are appropriate
- understand key concepts in monitoring vaccination programmes
- describe several important challenges in delivering vaccination
  programmes

Key terms

Adaptive immune system: Part of the overall immune system, which
develops throughout life as the body experiences different infections and
learns to recognize these.

Antibodies: Types of protein produced by the immune system that bind
precisely to an antigen to deactivate it.

Antigen: Any substance that causes an adaptive immune response.

Conjugation: A process used in the production of some vaccines in which the polysaccharide is chemically combined with a protein molecule.

Expanded Programme on Immunization (EPI):   A World Health Organization (WHO) programme introduced in 1974 that defines the vaccinations all countries should provide for their populations.

Herd effect: A reduced risk of infection among susceptible individuals owing to 'indirect protection' conferred by the presence and proximity of immune individuals in a population.

Herd immunity: When a sufficiently high proportion of the population is immune against a disease that the disease is unable to spread.

Immunization: The process by which a person is made immune from an infectious disease.

Mass vaccination: The administration of vaccines to a large population over a short period of time.

MMR: The combined measles, mumps and rubella triple vaccination.

Routine immunization: Administering vaccines for specified diseases to everybody at defined points in their life. Also known as universal immunization.

Targeted vaccination: The process of identifying people who are at elevated risk of a particular disease and targeting them for vaccination. Also known as selective vaccination.

Toxoids: Weakened toxins used in certain types of vaccines.

Vaccination: The process of administering a vaccine to a person or population with the aim of inducing immunity.

Vaccine: A biological preparation containing an antigenic substance that improves immunity to a particular disease.

The history of vaccination

Immunization is the process by which a person is made immune from an infectious disease. Vaccination is the process of administering a vaccine to a person or population with the aim of inducing immunity. These two terms are therefore closely related and often used interchangeably. One of the earliest known examples of vaccination dates back to the practice of variolation during the sixteenth century in China, which consisted of rubbing powdered scabs or fluids from smallpox pustules into superficial wounds in an uninfected person (Deng, 2011). Chapter 1 explained how this process became more widespread during the eighteenth century and the significant breakthroughs in vaccination made by Louis Pasteur in the second half of the nineteenth century. The word vaccination comes from *vaccinia*, the Latin word for cowpox, and was first used by Edward Jenner, who refined the practice of variolation in the eighteenth century. Many more vaccines were developed and introduced in the twentieth century, as shown in Figure 5.1.

In 1974, the WHO for the first time defined which vaccinations all countries worldwide should provide for their populations and developed resources to support countries to do so. This is known as the EPI. The aim of EPI is to ensure universal access to all relevant vaccines for all those at risk. At the time the EPI was introduced, it recommended the use of vaccines to protect against six diseases: tuberculosis (BCG), diphtheria, tetanus, pertussis (also known as whooping cough), measles and poliomyelitis.

In 2017, the WHO listed 26 diseases for which vaccines were available and a further 24 for which vaccines were in development (WHO, 2017). Immunization is one of the most powerful and cost-effective health interventions known (WHO, 2009). WHO data indicate that immunization prevents an estimated 2–3 million deaths every year from diphtheria, tetanus, pertussis and measles (WHO, 2016a). Figure 5.2 shows how immunizations have reduced cases of communicable diseases in India since 1975. However, almost 20 million children are not receiving routine immunization and an additional 1.5 million deaths every year could be avoided if global vaccination coverage were to improve (WHO, 2016a).

How vaccines work at the individual level: immunological concepts

Chapter 2 provided a brief explanation of how the immune system works. When an infectious agent enters the body, the immune system fights the infection. The adaptive immune system, which is one part of the overall immune system, develops throughout life as the body experiences different infections and learns to recognize these in order to fight them in the future. When the adaptive immune system recognizes an infectious agent and is able to neutralize it, the person is said to have immunity from the disease caused by the infectious agent. To fight infection, the immune system produces white blood cells, made up primarily of B-lymphocytes, T-lymphocytes and macrophages. Any substance that causes an adaptive immune response is known as an antigen. A vaccine carries an antigen that resembles the disease-causing microorganism and is often derived from attenuated forms of the microbe, its toxins or one of its surface proteins. This triggers an immune response without causing the actual disease. Once injected the antigen, which is contained in the vaccine, is enveloped by an antigen-presenting complex (APC). The APC interacts with immune

Historical vaccine development and introduction of routine vaccine programmes in the UK

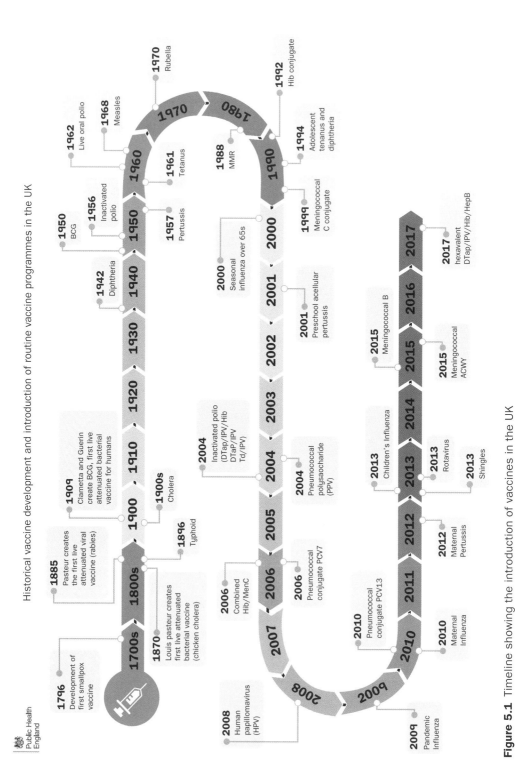

Figure 5.1 Timeline showing the introduction of vaccines in the UK

Source: Public Health England (2017).

VACCINES WORK: INDIA

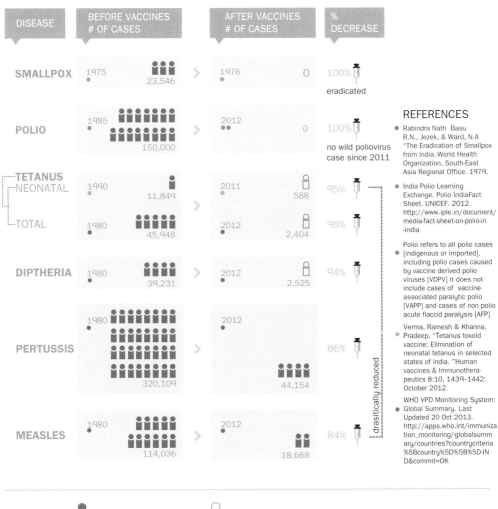

DISEASE	BEFORE VACCINES # OF CASES	AFTER VACCINES # OF CASES	% DECREASE
SMALLPOX	1975 — 23,546	1976 — 0	100% eradicated
POLIO	1985 — 150,000	2012 — 0	100% no wild poliovirus case since 2011
TETANUS NEONATAL	1990 — 11,849	2011 — 588	95%
TETANUS TOTAL	1980 — 45,948	2012 — 2,404	95%
DIPTHERIA	1980 — 39,231	2012 — 2,525	94%
PERTUSSIS	1980 — 320,109	2012 — 44,154	86%
MEASLES	1980 — 114,036	2012 — 18,668	84%

REFERENCES

- Rabindra Nath Basu R.N., Jezek, & Ward, N.A "The Eradication of Smallpox from India.-World Health Organization, South-East Asia Regional Office. 1979.

- India Polio Learning Exchange. Polio IndiaFact Sheet. UNICEF. 2012. http://www.iple.in/document/media-fact-sheet-on-polio-in-india

- Polio refers to all polio cases [indigenous or imported], including polio cases caused by vaccine derived polio viruses [VDPV] it does not include cases of vaccine-associated paralytic polio [VAPP] and cases of non polio acute flaccid paralysis [AFP]

- Verma, Ramesh & Khanna, Pradeep, "Tetanus toxoid vaccine: Elimination of neonatal tetanus in selected states of india. "Human vaccines & Immunotherapeutics 8:10, 1439–1442: October 2012.

- WHO VPD Monitoring System: Global Summary. Last Updated 20 Oct 2013. http://apps.who.int/immunization_monitoring/globalsummary/countries?countrycriteria%5Bcountry%5D%5B%5D-IND&commit=OK

drastically reduced

🔹 10,000 reported cases 🔹 Less than 10,000 reported cases

Figure 5.2 The impact of vaccines in India

Source: International Vaccines Access Center, Johns Hopkins University (2013).

components known as CD4 and CD8 cells that are types of T-lymphocytes. This interaction causes a cascade of cell production, which, after a period of around a few weeks, results in the development of 'memory' cells. These memory cells enable the immune system to identify and better respond to the antigen the vaccine introduced the next time it enters. It does so by producing antibodies, which are types of protein that bind precisely to an antigen to deactivate it. This means if the infectious agent targeted by the vaccine enters the body, the immune system will produce antibodies specially tailored to bind to that specific antigen, thus neutralizing the threat it presents. Sources of more detailed information about how vaccination works can be found in the further reading section at the end of this chapter.

Different types of vaccine

Different types of vaccine are administered in different ways. The type that is used depends on the disease. For some diseases, there are several potential vaccines and which one is used depends on the particular strain of the disease, the health status of the person being vaccinated, logistical factors and availability. Vaccines are classified into two main groups, live attenuated vaccines and inactivated vaccines, which are then further subdivided, as illustrated in Table 5.1. An additional type of vaccine, recombinant vaccines, has been recently developed. Understanding the main types of vaccines and their key features is important for designing vaccination strategies. These are described below.

Live attenuated vaccines

Live attenuated vaccines are produced by modifying a 'wild' disease-causing virus or bacterium in a laboratory to produce a weakened or 'attenuated' form. This is usually done by repeated culturing. A relatively small dose of the attenuated virus or bacteria is given as a vaccine. This attenuated virus or bacteria then multiplies in the vaccinated individual, increasing the quantity of antigen and producing immunity. Although it usually does not cause illness, in some cases it can produce symptoms that are much

Table 5.1 Classification of vaccines

Live attenuated vaccines	• Viral
	• Bacterial
Inactivated vaccines	• Whole
	◦ Viruses
	◦ Bacteria
	• Fractional
	◦ Protein-based
	▪ Toxoid
	▪ Subunit
	◦ Polysaccharide-based
	▪ Pure
	▪ Conjugate

Source: CDC (2015).

milder than the actual disease. Live attenuated vaccines are subdivided into viral and bacterial vaccines. The majority of live attenuated vaccines are used for viruses: MMR, varicella, yellow fever and influenza. Bacterial live vaccines are available for TB and typhoid.

Live vaccines have the advantage of producing an immune response that is virtually identical to that produced by the actual disease. Usually, they only need to be given as a single dose to be effective. However, they do have some disadvantages. Because they are live, changes in temperature and light can harm them, so they must be handled and stored carefully. They may cause severe or even fatal reactions as a result of uncontrolled growth of the virus in the vaccine in immunosuppressed individuals, such as people with leukaemia, those with low CD4 counts due to HIV, or people undergoing certain forms of medical treatment like chemotherapy. A live attenuated vaccine virus can also revert to its original form and cause disease, although this is only known to happen with the live oral polio vaccine. Finally, active immunity from a live attenuated vaccine may not develop due to interference from circulating antibodies from another source, such as a young baby who still has some immunity from their mother or someone who has recently received antibody-containing blood products at the time the vaccine is given, which can lead to vaccine failure.

Despite these limitations, live vaccines against viral diseases are one of the most cost-effective health interventions currently available. Their use has eradicated smallpox and is likely to eradicate polio in the near future. Measles has also been controlled in the Western hemisphere and in much of the developing world. New live attenuated vaccines against rotavirus may be the best way to reduce rotavirus mortality (Minor, 2015).

Inactivated vaccines

Inactivated vaccines are made by growing the bacteria or virus and then inactivating or killing them with heat and/or chemicals. Inactivated vaccines produce immune responses in different ways than live attenuated vaccines. Inactivated vaccines are not alive and so the antigen cannot replicate after it is injected. Therefore, the entire dose of antigen is administered in the vaccination. Multiple doses are necessary to build up and maintain immunity. In general, the first dose does not produce protective immunity. A protective immune response develops after the second or third dose. Immunity from inactivated vaccines also usually diminishes with time. As a result, some inactivated vaccines may require periodic supplemental doses to top up or 'boost' immunity. Unlike live attenuated vaccines, inactivated vaccines cannot cause disease, even in an immune-deficient person and they are usually not affected by circulating antibodies so they may be given when antibodies are present in the blood. Inactivated vaccines can be easily stored and transported in a freeze-dried form because they are not alive, which makes the organization of vaccination campaigns easier where infrastructure is weak and stable temperatures are difficult to maintain. However, because several doses and boosters are required, follow-up vaccination is needed, which can be a limitation where there are no routine vaccination services. Inactivated vaccines are divided into whole inactivated and fractional inactivated vaccines:

Whole inactivated vaccines

Whole inactivated vaccines are made from using whole viruses and bacteria that are inactivated by chemicals or heat. Whole inactivated vaccines for viruses include polio, rabies, hepatitis A and influenza; and whole inactivated vaccines for bacteria, include pertussis, typhoid, cholera and plague.

Fractional inactivated vaccines

Fractional inactivated vaccines are inactivated vaccines made from pieces of bacteria or viruses. Fractional inactivated vaccines are divided into two groups: protein-based and polysaccharide-based.

- *Protein-based vaccines*: Protein-based vaccines include toxoid vaccines and subunit vaccines. Toxoid vaccines prevent diseases caused by toxins produced by bacteria. They are made by weakening a toxin so it cannot cause illness. Weakened toxins are called toxoids. When the immune system receives a vaccine containing a toxoid, it learns how to fight off the natural toxin. It does so by producing antibodies that lock onto and block the toxin. Examples include the diphtheria and tetanus vaccines. Subunit vaccines are made from pieces of viruses or bacteria that are selected because they are able to stimulate the immune system without causing disease. Currently available inactivated subunit vaccines include hepatitis B, human papillomavirus, inactivated influenza, acellular pertussis, anthrax and Lyme disease.
- *Polysaccharide-based vaccines*: Polysaccharide vaccines are composed of long chains of sugar molecules that make up the surface capsule of certain bacteria. The immune response to a pure polysaccharide vaccine is typically T-cell independent, which means that these vaccines are able to stimulate B cells without the assistance of T-helper cells. Polysaccharide vaccines include pneumococcal, meningococcal and typhoid Vi. However, T-cell-independent antigens, including polysaccharide vaccines, do not consistently cause immunity in children younger than 2 years of age because of immaturity of the immune system. Also, repeated doses of polysaccharide vaccine do not usually boost immunity. In the late 1980s, it was discovered that these limitations could be overcome through a process called conjugation, in which the polysaccharide is chemically combined with a protein molecule. Conjugation changes the immune response from T-cell independent to T-cell dependent, leading to increased immunogenicity in infants and antibody booster response to multiple doses of

vaccine. Currently available conjugate vaccines include *Haemophilus influenzae* type b, meningococcal and pneumococcal vaccines (CDC, 2015).

Recombinant vaccines

Recombinant vaccines are a newer type of vaccine involving antigens that are produced by genetic engineering technology. Genetically engineered vaccines that are currently available include hepatitis B, human papillomavirus and influenza. Recombinant vaccine technology is rapidly developing using different approaches to stimulate the immune system. These include using live recombinant bacteria or viral vectors, DNA vaccines and prime-boost strategies combining different antigen delivery systems to broaden the immune response (Nascimento and Leite, 2012).

How vaccines work at the population level: herd immunity and the basic reproduction number

Vaccines for communicable diseases do not work at the level of the individual alone. The presence of immune individuals in a population can also reduce the risk of infection among susceptible (non-immune) individuals, through what is known as a 'herd effect'. If immunization coverage rate is high, this herd effect can produce what is known as 'herd immunity' for some communicable diseases. Herd immunity occurs when a sufficiently high proportion of the population is immune against a disease, either from having been infected or from having been vaccinated so that the disease is unable to spread because there are so few susceptible people left to infect. The minimum proportion of a population that must be immune in order to achieve herd immunity is referred to as the herd immunity threshold (Fine *et al.*, 2011).

The herd immunity threshold varies between diseases, and between settings for a given disease, depending on what is known as the basic reproduction number, often referred to as R_0 (pronounced 'R-naught' or 'R-zero'). The basic reproduction number is defined as the average number of secondary cases caused by a single infected case in an otherwise susceptible population. The basic reproductive number of an infectious disease can be expressed as:

$$R_0 = \beta \times N \times D$$

where β is the probability of transmitting the infection for each contact, N is the contact rate (i.e. the average number of people an individual comes into contact with over a given period of time) and D is the duration of the infectious period. When R_0 is less than 1, each infected person will cause, on average, less than one new infected person and the infection will not survive in the population. Where R_0 is greater than 1, each infected person will cause, on average, more than one new infected person and therefore the infection will spread.

R_0 essentially represents the maximum transmission potential of a disease when it is introduced into a previously unexposed population, because it assumes that all the contacts of an infected case are susceptible individuals. However, as the proportion of infected and immune people increases, so too does the likelihood that some of those contacts will already be infected or immune. The net case reproduction number, R, represents actual transmission in a population taking into account the proportion of individuals that are immune at a given time. It is calculated using the following equation:

$R = R_0(1 - p)$

where p is the proportion of the population that is immune (either through natural immunity, because they were infected, or because they have been vaccinated). When R is greater than 1, the disease will continue to spread and an epidemic may occur. If $R = 1$, the disease remains at a steady endemic state. But if R becomes less than 1, the disease will die out. So, using the equation above, we can show that herd immunity is achieved if:

$R_0(1 - p) < 1$

Rearranging this formula allows us to estimate the herd immunity threshold for a disease based on its R_0:

$p > 1 - (1/R_0)$

R_0 varies for different diseases. Measles, for example, is highly contagious with R_0 estimates typically ranging from 12 to 18. In a population where measles has an R_0 of 16, the above equation gives a herd immunity threshold of $> 1 - (1/16)$, so $p > 0.94$. In other words, at least 94% of the population needs to be immune to achieve herd immunity and eliminate transmission. For polio, which is less contagious with an R_0 of around 5–7, around 80% to 86% of the population must be immunized. However, when immunization rates fall, herd immunity can break down leading to an increase in the number of new cases. Herd immunity is important because it means that disease elimination is possible with less than 100% immunization coverage in a population. In any community there will always be some people who cannot be immunized against a disease, for example because they are immunosuppressed due to another illness.

Activity 5.1

What do you think would be the consequences of a fall in the vaccination coverage rate for a communicable disease? If there is very low incidence of a certain communicable disease, is it safe to stop vaccinating against it and use the resources for another aspect of health care?

Feedback

If vaccination coverage rates are not maintained at a sufficiently high level to ensure herd immunity, an epidemic of a communicable disease can quickly take hold. This is the case even if the incidence of that disease has previously fallen to very low levels. Unless a disease has been eradicated, as in the case of smallpox, vaccination needs to continue. An example from Japan relates to pertussis. In 1974, about 80% of Japanese children were receiving pertussis vaccine. There were only 393 cases of pertussis in the entire country and not a single pertussis-related death in that year. Immunization rates then began to decrease until only about 10% of children were being vaccinated. Then, in 1979, there were more than 13,000 cases of pertussis and 41 died as a result. When routine vaccination was resumed, cases of pertussis reduced again (CDC, 2017).

Vaccination strategies

The aim of all vaccination strategies is to meet disease reduction goals by achieving high levels of immunity in the targeted population through adequate immunization coverage and vaccine effectiveness (Hardt *et al.*, 2016). Different strategies are used to achieve this aim depending on such factors as the disease in question and type of vaccination available, the target population for vaccination, local healthcare infrastructure, funding, existing vaccination coverage and the availability of vaccines. The main strategies are routine immunization, mass vaccination campaigns and targeted vaccination campaigns. Vaccination is also sometimes used for people travelling to countries, or areas within a country, where diseases not covered by their home country's routine immunization programmes are endemic. The main vaccination strategies are now described in more detail.

Routine immunization

Most vaccinations take place through routine immunization services and are delivered through existing healthcare services as part of on-going health care. In some contexts, routine immunization is known as universal immunization. This involves administering vaccines for specified diseases to everybody at defined points in their life. Most are given during infancy and childhood and they take the EPI described earlier as their starting point. Since the introduction of the EPI in 1974, the WHO has added vaccinations to the recommended schedule. The WHO now recommends that all countries provide vaccinations against the hepatitis B virus, *Haemophilus influenzae* type b, pneumococcus, rotavirus, rubella virus and human papillomavirus, in addition to the original six diseases covered by the EPI (tuberculosis,

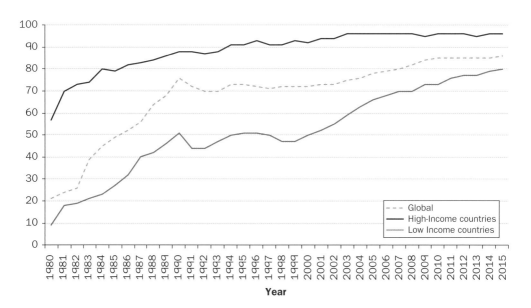

Figure 5.3 Coverage with three doses of diphtheria-, tetanus- and pertussis-containing vaccines (DTP3), by country income levels, 1980–2015

Source: WHO/UNICEF coverage estimates 2015 revision. July 2016 and Country Income Categories (World Bank) as of July 2016 (2015 GNI per capita).

diphtheria, tetanus, pertussis, measles and poliomyelitis). There are additional recommendations for certain countries and population groups at risk of specific diseases. The EPI schedule is updated regularly by the WHO to take account of new vaccines and is available on the WHO website. Most countries adapt the EPI by adding additional vaccinations that the health authorities there consider to be needed based on local conditions and availability. In some countries, certain childhood vaccinations are mandatory and parents may be prosecuted if they refuse to have their children vaccinated. In other countries, vaccinations are not mandatory but are strongly recommended. Some countries also offer financial incentives to parents to have their children vaccinated (Walkinshaw, 2011).

The number of countries achieving coverage according to at least some of the EPI recommendations has increased dramatically since 1980, as Figure 5.3 shows. However, in 2015, an estimated 19.4 million infants worldwide were still not receiving routine immunization services such as the diphtheria, tetanus and pertussis vaccine and around 1.5 million deaths could have been prevented through higher vaccination coverage. The WHO has identified five factors necessary for achieving widespread immunization coverage:

- Quality and use of data
- Community involvement

- Better access to immunization services for marginalized and displaced populations
- Strong health systems
- Access to vaccines in all places at all times (WHO, 2016a).

The advantages of routine immunization programmes include: they can be incorporated into regular healthcare services; they aim to cover the entire population; they are generally good at achieving herd immunity; and they may be more likely to be accepted by the public because everybody is subject to them. Disadvantages include they can be costly and they are not appropriate for all vaccines, due to factors such as potential side-effects or the need for complicated administration.

Mass vaccination campaigns

A mass vaccination campaign involves the administration of vaccines to a large population over a short period of time. Mass vaccination campaigns can target an entire population in an affected area or a population group at increased risk. Mass vaccination campaigns are typically undertaken for several reasons. First, mass vaccination campaigns may be undertaken in response to an emerging epidemic in order to stop the epidemic spreading. The aim of a mass vaccination campaign in this circumstance is to rapidly limit morbidity and mortality from a vaccine-preventable disease that has been confirmed by increasing the immunity of the population. One example is the use of mass vaccination to prevent the spread of cholera (Ciglenecki et al., 2013). Another example is mass vaccination against yellow fever (see Activity 5.2).

Second, mass vaccination may be undertaken in response to the threat of an epidemic that has not yet been established. The aim of a mass vaccination campaign here is to establish population immunity before the disease epidemic starts. This is an approach that is used in areas where diseases are endemic and/or at high risk of causing an epidemic, for example, mass vaccination campaigns against typhoid fever (Yang et al., 2005). Mass vaccination campaigns to prevent epidemics are often used in humanitarian emergencies such as conflict, natural disasters, food insecurity or other crises, as there may be low levels of pre-existing population immunity and the displacement and poor living conditions of the population are likely to increase the risk of an outbreak. In particular, evidence suggests that in such situations vaccinating all children aged 6 months to 15 years against measles is warranted (Grais et al., 2011).

Third, mass vaccination campaigns can be used when national routine immunization coverage rates are not sufficient to generate herd immunity. These are often known as 'catch-up' campaigns. Their aim is to bring vaccination rates up to the target level of routine immunization programmes. Catch-up campaigns have been used when vaccination coverage rates in routine immunization programmes have fallen during a specific time period.

For example, in 2013 a MMR vaccination catch-up campaign was under-taken in England and Wales, which targeted around one million children, born between 1997 and 2003, who were unvaccinated or only partially vacci-nated against measles as a result of the controversy about the safety of the MMR vaccine (NHS Choices, 2013). Catch-up campaigns are frequently used in low-income countries where healthcare and public health infra-structure is under-developed and routine immunization programmes do not achieve adequate coverage (Babu *et al.*, 2012). They are also sometimes used when a new vaccine is being introduced. In this case, catch-up immuni-zation for older age groups may be used together with routine immunization for infants or young children. This approach can rapidly reduce transmission of a disease. In general, new vaccines should be incorporated into routine immunization programmes as soon as possible in order to minimize disrup-tion (WHO, 2012).

Finally, mass vaccination campaigns are used as part of disease eradica-tion programmes. As discussed in Chapter 1, the global campaign for smallpox eradication used a strategy of mass vaccination campaigns, supple-mented with aggressive case-finding and vaccination of all possible contacts where mass vaccination was not achievable. Supplementary immunization activities (SIAs) have been a key strategy of the Global Polio Eradication Initiative (GPEI). SIAs are mass vaccination campaigns that aim to administer additional doses of oral poliovirus vaccine to children aged 5 years or under, regardless of whether they may already have been vaccinated. In many countries, SIAs have made a substantial contribution to the 99% global reduction in the incidence of paralytic poliomyelitis that has been achieved since the launch of the GPEI in 1988 (Helleringer *et al.*, 2012).

The advantages of mass vaccination campaigns include that the urgency they imply may convince people they should get vaccinated, they can establish herd immunity quickly and they can contain a disease and prevent it spreading. Their disadvantages are that they can cause panic and backlash, they can be difficult to organize logistically and they are costly.

Whatever their specific objective, mass vaccination campaigns involve considerable planning, resources and logistical support because large numbers of people are being vaccinated in a short period of time. Particular consideration is needed to:

• secure financial and other resources well in advance;
• plan for the campaign at the right time of year, including factors such as when people are likely to be available (such as during school holiday), avoiding months when weather is most likely to be unfavourable and before the next peak in incidence is expected;
• ensure that there are enough supplies of vaccines and syringes (unless it is an oral vaccine);
• maintain the right temperature – if the campaign relies on a live vaccine, this may require the use of thousands of ice packs and portable refrigerators with the required power to maintain the cold chain;

- ensure there are sufficient human resources for vaccine administration – this may require training people who are not health professionals to administer vaccines;
- provide facilities for the safe disposal of used syringes and needles;
- provide transportation for the vaccination teams and vaccines, including to areas that may be hard to reach;
- undertake communication, community engagement and social mobilization so that the affected communities are aware of the campaign and understand its importance.

Poorly planned or poorly implemented mass campaigns can result in the waste of scarce resources and generate suspicion of future vaccination activities among the population.

Targeted vaccination campaigns

Another vaccination strategy involves identifying people who are at elevated risk of particular disease and targeting them for vaccination. This is known as targeted or selective vaccination. One example of this is the influenza vaccine. The WHO recommends that healthcare workers and people who have a higher risk of medical complications from flu be vaccinated. These include pregnant women, people with certain chronic diseases, older people and residents of institutions. This strategy is used because most healthy adults have a very low risk of complications from influenza infection, and vaccine supplies are generally limited because the vaccines need to be updated annually to respond to changes in flu strains. Another example is targeting teenagers and students starting university for the first time for a vaccination to prevent meningitis W disease. This is because they are at high risk of infection due to high rates of social mixing between lots of new people (NHS Choices, 2016).

The advantages of targeted vaccination include that it can be more cost-effective and efficient than a mass campaign, it limits exposure to unnecessary side-effects in most of the population, and it conserves resources and healthcare workers' time. The disadvantages are that it does not generate herd immunity and some individuals in the target group may be missed.

Vaccinations for individuals planning to travel

In addition to the vaccination strategies described in this section, when individuals travel away from their own countries they may require extra vaccinations. This can be viewed as a type of selective or targeted vaccination. This is usually the case if they are visiting countries that are endemic for diseases not included in their home countries' routine immunization programmes. Common vaccinations required for travel to some countries include Japanese encephalitis and tick-borne encephalitis, meningitis, rabies, tuberculosis, yellow fever, typhoid, hepatitis A, hepatitis B and cholera. Some countries with a high risk of yellow fever transmission require a certificate to prove the person has been vaccinated against the condition before they are allowed entry. The certificate is known as an International Certificate of Vaccination or Prophylaxis (ICVP). Some countries make certain travel vaccinations available free as part of the healthcare provision because there is a recognized public health benefit in minimizing the risk of people returning home infected with a communicable disease. Other countries see this as the responsibility of the individual who is planning to travel. The authorities may provide advice through the public health system but require individuals to arrange vaccinations themselves and pay for these in private clinics.

✎ Activity 5.2

Yellow fever is an acute viral haemorrhagic disease transmitted by infected mosquitoes. The 'yellow' in the name refers to the jaundice that affects some patients. Case fatality rates for reported cases range from around 15% to 50%. It is endemic in some tropical areas of Africa and Central and South America. Large epidemics of yellow fever occur when infected people introduce the virus into heavily populated areas with high mosquito density and where most people have little or no immunity, due to lack of vaccination. An extremely effective live vaccine is available, which is safe, affordable and only requires one dose. In 2016, an outbreak affected people in urban areas of Angola and the Democratic Republic of the Congo. What type of vaccination campaign do you think is required, and why? What do you think are the logistical requirements of such a campaign?

Feedback

A yellow fever outbreak like this requires a mass vaccination campaign, given the severity of the disease and the availability of an effective vaccine. Logistical considerations you might have reflected on include: a large number of people will need to be vaccinated as the outbreak threatens urban areas which are densely populated; large numbers of vaccines and syringes will be needed; lots of people will need to be recruited to administer the vaccine and provide logistical support; these people will require training; the vaccine is live so it will need to be kept at the right temperature in a tropical area, which will require appropriate storage facilities such as gas-, solar- or electric-powered refrigerators at the main clinic/hospital and cool boxes and vaccine carriers for

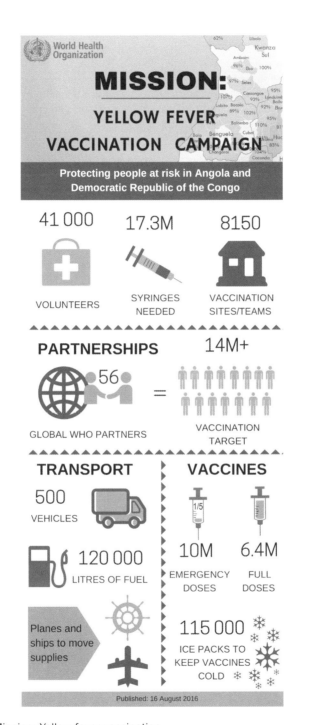

Figure 5.4 WHO Mission: Yellow fever vaccination
Source: WHO (2016c).

transporting vaccines to community clinics; the vaccines will need to be transported and road infrastructure may be poor; the community will need to be engaged in advance so they understand the importance of vaccination. More information on this vaccination campaign can be seen in the infographic in Figure 5.4.

Surveillance of vaccination programmes

Surveillance related to vaccine-preventable diseases is an essential part of communicable disease surveillance, as discussed in the previous chapter. It is used to:

- monitor vaccination coverage rates so as to identify if these are falling, enabling action to be taken before they reach levels where outbreaks may become possible;
- identify trends in disease incidence that may indicate a vaccination or a vaccination strategy is not working as planned;
- identify if there are any population groups that are not being adequately reached by vaccination activities;
- inform the management of vaccine supply;
- monitor the effectiveness of new vaccines;
- monitor adverse reactions to new vaccines and develop information to respond to any safety concerns among the public;
- identify any areas where routine immunization programmes may need re-enforcing;
- monitor progress towards specific goals, for example polio eradication and measles control or elimination;
- inform policy-making on vaccination strategies.

In addition to the epidemiological concepts involved in communicable disease surveillance that the last chapter introduced, the surveillance and evaluation of vaccination programmes includes some specific measures:

- *Vaccination coverage rates*: The vaccination coverage rate is the percentage of the targeted population that has been vaccinated against a disease. Routine immunization needs to achieve good coverage to be effective.
- *Vaccine efficacy*: The reduction in disease incidence in a vaccinated group compared with an unvaccinated group. Vaccine efficacy is best measured by double-blind, randomized, clinical controlled trials. Vaccine efficacy trials represent the 'best case scenarios' of vaccine protectiveness under controlled conditions and are commonly required before a new vaccine is licensed. The outcome data are generally expressed as a proportionate reduction in disease attack rate between the unvacci-

nated and vaccinated study cohorts (Weinberg and Szilagy, 2010). Vaccine efficacy is generally measured in controlled vaccine trials, rather than as part of routine vaccine surveillance.

- *Vaccine effectiveness*: A 'real world' view of how a vaccine, which may have already proven to have high vaccine efficacy, reduces disease in a population in natural conditions, as opposed to a controlled clinical trial. Vaccine effectiveness is proportional to vaccine efficacy but is also affected by other factors, including how well target groups are immunized and non-vaccine-related factors (Weinberg and Szilagy, 2010).

- *Vaccine impact*: This is a broader measure that involves evaluating the direct effects on vaccinated individuals and the indirect effects on the unvaccinated community through herd immunity, the prevention of transmission and additional benefits resulting from improved health (Doherty *et al.*, 2016).

- *Adverse events following immunization*: These are untoward medical occurrences that follow vaccination, sometimes known as a vaccine adverse events. Although all vaccines must be proven safe and effective before they are licensed, no vaccine is completely risk-free and adverse events will occasionally result after a vaccination. An adverse event may be any unfavourable or unintended sign, abnormal laboratory finding, symptom or disease. It does not necessarily have a causal relationship with the usage of the vaccine. Adverse events need to be reported and investigated carefully and transparently to ensure public trust in vaccination is maintained. International and national reporting systems are in place to do this, including the Vaccine Adverse Event Reporting System (VAERS) in the USA (CDC, 2012).

Vaccination challenges

Vaccines have saved hundreds of millions of lives and are widely acknowledged to be one of the greatest medical developments of all time (Worboys, 2007). However, despite these achievements and a century after widespread vaccination against common communicable diseases was introduced, several important challenges in the development and delivery of vaccination programmes remain.

First, as this book goes on to discuss in Chapter 11, new and emerging infectious diseases present a growing threat. For example, an outbreak of Ebola virus disease (EVD) in West Africa that began in 2014 resulted in the deaths of over 11,000 people, left over 17,300 children as orphans, caused huge economic and social disruption, and severely disrupted the provision of health care including treatment and control of HIV, tuberculosis and malaria (CDC, 2016). However, at the time of the outbreak no vaccine existed for EVD. Vaccine development typically takes more than 10 years. This means leadership, funding and systems must be in place to rapidly fast track the development of vaccines for new infectious diseases as they emerge. A new international initiative, the Coalition for Epidemic Prepared-ness Innovations (CEPI), has recently been established with this goal in mind (CEPI, 2017).

Second, good vaccination coverage requires routine immunization programmes that are effective and embedded in the healthcare system. However, in some countries these routine immunization programmes lack sufficient resources and support. In addition, research indicates that in some countries the addition of new vaccinations to the EPI has placed increased stress on routine immunization programmes (Steinglass, 2013). The cost of the EPI has also increased significantly as more vacci-nations have been included. Immunization budgets in many low- and low-to-middle-income countries are currently insufficient (Shen *et al.*, 2014). As will be discussed in Chapter 10, healthcare systems in many low- and low-to-middle-income countries are under-resourced and lack adequate infrastructure, trained staff and leadership. Rural communities are often particularly under-served, with healthcare infrastructure better serving urban areas. In addition, logistical requirements for transporting and storing vaccines at refrigerated temperatures can present considerable difficulties. The introduction of new and more expensive vaccines that are at risk of damage from heat and/or freeze exposure has made this even more significant. The importance of developing vaccines with improved thermo-stability has been recognized by vaccine developers and other stakeholders (Kristensen *et al.*, 2016). A lack of resources and infrastruc-ture for routine immunization contributes to the failure to ensure that all children have access to the recommended vaccinations, resulting in around 1.5 million deaths that could have been avoided with full coverage (WHO, 2016b).

A third challenge, that the vaccine must be acceptable to the population, is essential to achieve the required level of coverage. Vaccines are differ-ent from other forms of medications because they are given to healthy individuals, usually children, to prevent diseases that often are not seen as posing an immediate threat. Controversy about vaccine safety can cause parents to decide the potential risks of a vaccination outweigh the potential benefits, which can result in falls in vaccination coverage rates. Accept-ability is influenced by many factors, including trust of healthcare workers, newspaper reports, the views of other family members and friends, and whether vaccination is compulsory. Research has shown parents may give too much weight to the perceived risks of the vaccination and not enough to the risks of their child getting the disease and becoming seriously ill. Surveys have shown that there is wide variability between countries and across world regions as to confidence in vaccine safety, and it is particu-larly low in the European region (The Vaccine Confidence Project, 2016).

One example of how public confidence in a vaccine can influence take-up is the MMR controversy that followed the publication of an article in *The Lancet* in 1998 by Andrew Wakefield, in which a link was suggested between the MMR vaccine and autism. The research behind the article was subsequently shown to be flawed and the article was retracted (*The Lancet*, 2010). However, it generated huge media coverage, which contributed to changes in parental attitudes towards the MMR vaccine and a loss of trust in healthcare services. This resulted in a decline in uptake. For example, the number of children in Scotland vaccinated by their second birthday fell from almost 95% in 1997 to 87% in 2001 (Allan and Harden, 2015).

 Activity 5.3

Take a look at Table 5.2, which details cases of MMR in England and Wales from 1996 to 2012. Cases in England only are shown in brackets. What trends can you identify? What do you think the reasons might be?

Table 5.2 Confirmed cases of MMR in England and Wales (England only in parentheses), 1996–2012

	Measles	Mumps	Rubella
1996	112 (112)	94 (93)	3922 (3567)
1997	177 (177)	182 (172)	117 (113)
1998	56 (55)	121 (118)	119 (117)
1999	92 (92)	373 (371)	162 (159)
2000	100 (99)	730 (721)	62 (61)
2001	70 (67)	784 (731)	45 (41)
2002	319 (316)	500 (394)	64 (64)
2003	437 (393)	1541 (1086)	16 (14)
2004	188 (178)	8129 (7321)	14 (14)
2005	78 (78)	43378 (39621)	29 (27)
2006	740 (736)	4420 (4128)	34 (34)
2007	990 (977)	1476 (1462)	35 (35)
2008	1370 (1331)	2405 (2348)	27 (27)
2009	1144 (985)	7662 (7301)	9 (9)
2010	380 (372)	3965 (3880)	12 (12)
2011	1087 (1068)	2372 (2299)	6 (6)
2012	2030 (1912)	2564 (2476)	65 (65)

Source: Public Health England, http://webarchive.nationalarchives.gov.uk/20140505192923/http:/www.hpa.org.uk/web/HPAweb&HPAweb-Standard/HPAweb_C/1195733833790.

Feedback

You should have noticed that after 2001 cases of measles began to rise, with identifiable outbreaks. This is because there was a sharp fall in the vaccination coverage rate from the late 1990s onwards, resulting in immunization rates below the level required for herd immunity, as illustrated in Figure 5.5. The measles, mumps and rubella triple vaccine (MMR) was introduced in the UK in 1988. In February 1998, a paper suggesting a link between the MMR vaccine and autism and bowel symptoms was published in the highly respected British medical journal *The Lancet*. Although the research described in the article was subsequently proven to be flawed and was withdrawn (as described above), the controversy the article provoked was widely reported and contributed to some parents deciding not to get their children vaccinated (Casiday et al., 2006).

You should also have noticed that there was a major epidemic of mumps in 2004/05. MMR vaccination of 1-year-olds was started in 1988, coinciding with a preschool catch-up programme. Mumps became notifiable in England and Wales at that time, and its incidence fell drastically during the 1990s. However, small outbreaks of measles occurred in children at secondary school in the early 1990s that prompted a national

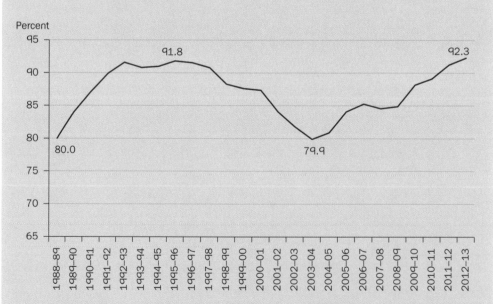

Figure 5.5 Coverage of the measles, mumps and rubella (MMR) vaccine in England for children reaching their second birthday

Source: NHS Immunization Statistics (HSCIC, 2013) England 2012–13. Copyright © 2013 HSCIC, http://content.digital.nhs.uk/catalogue/PUB11665/nhs-immu-stat-eng-2012-13-rep.pdf.

catch-up campaign for 5–16-year-olds in 1994. Instead of the MMR vaccine, combined measles and rubella preparation was used. This was because of a shortage of mumps vaccine and the MMR vaccine at the time. The 2004/05 outbreak affected in particular individuals born between 1982 and 1986 that had neither been previously exposed to natural infection (due to the reduction in circulating mumps) nor protected by vaccination because they had not received MMR. Around 98% of people born before 1982 are immune, owing to natural infection in the pre-MMR era (Gupta *et al.*, 2005).

You might have noticed that rubella cases did not rise in the same way. The fact that rubella is less easily transmitted than measles and, therefore, requires a lower rate of vaccination coverage for herd immunity may explain this.

Summary

Vaccination against common communicable diseases is a safe, highly effective and cost-effective intervention. Approximately 26 diseases are vaccine-preventable. New vaccines and new approaches to vaccine development based on emerging technologies offer the potential that more diseases could be prevented in the near future. However, vaccination does not offer a permanent or easy solution for communicable disease control. Providing universal access across the world to the required vaccinations continues to be very challenging. Healthcare systems in low-income countries may lack the capacity to provide routine immunization in line with the EPI. In addition, unless vaccination coverage rates are maintained at a high level, disease control can rapidly break down, leading to renewed epidemics. Public acceptability of vaccination, which is influenced by many factors, is crucial. The next chapter turns to the other strategies that can be used to prevent outbreaks and control communicable disease, in addition to vaccination. These are especially important for diseases where vaccination is not possible.

Further reading

Siegrist, C.A. (2013) Vaccine immunology, in S. Plotkin, W. Orenstein and P. Offit (eds.) *Vaccines*, 6th edn. (pp. 14–32). Philadelphia, PA: Elsevier Health Sciences

References

Allan, N. and Harden, J. (2015) Parental decision-making in uptake of the MMR vaccination: a systematic review of qualitative literature, *Journal of Public Health (Oxford)*, 37 (4): 678–687.

Babu, G.R., Sathyanarayana, T.N., Jana, S., Nandy, S., Farid, M.N. and Sadhana, S.M. (2012) Role of catch-up campaigns in improving immunization services in a developing country, *Annals of Tropical Medicine and Public Health*, 5 (5): 441–446.

Casiday, R., Cresswell, T., Wilson, D. and Panter-Brick, C. (2006) A survey of UK parental attitudes to the MMR vaccine and trust in medical authority, *Vaccine*, 24 (2): 177–184.

Centers for Disease Control and Prevention (CDC) (2012) *Understanding the Vaccine Adverse Event Reporting System (VAERS)*. Available at: https://www.cdc.gov/vaccines/hcp/patient-ed/conversations/downloads/vacsafe-vaers-color-office.pdf [accessed 9 March 2017].

Centers for Disease Control and Prevention (CDC) (2015) *Epidemiology and Prevention of Vaccine-Preventable Diseases*, 13th edn. Washington, DC: Public Health Foundation.

Centers for Disease Control and Prevention (CDC) (2016) *Cost of the Ebola epidemic*. Available at: https://www.cdc.gov/vhf/ebola/outbreaks/2014-west-africa/cost-of-ebola.html [accessed 9 March 2017].

Centers for Disease Control and Prevention (CDC) (2017) *What would happen if we stopped vaccinations?* Available at: https://www.cdc.gov/vaccines/vac-gen/whatifstop.htm [accessed 9 March 2017].

Ciglenecki, I., Sakoba, K., Luquero, F.J., Heile, M., Itama, C., Mengel, M. *et al.* (2013) Feasibility of mass vaccination campaign with oral cholera vaccines in response to an outbreak in Guinea, *PLoS Medicine*, 10 (9): e1001512.

Coalition for Epidemic Preparedness Innovations (CEPI) (2017) *New vaccines for a safer world*. Available at: http://cepi.net/sites/default/files/CEPI_2pager_16_Feb_17.pdf [accessed 9 March 2017].

Deng, Y. (2011) *Ancient Chinese Inventions*. Cambridge: Cambridge University Press.

Doherty, M., Buchy, P., Standaert, B., Giaquinto, C. and Prado-Cohrs, D. (2016) Vaccine impact: benefits for human health, *Vaccine*, 34 (52): 6707–6714.

Fine, P., Eames, K. and Heymann, D.L. (2011) Herd immunity: a rough guide, *Clinical Infectious Diseases*, 52: 911–916.

Grais, R.F., Strebel, P., Mala, P., Watson, J., Nandy, R. and Gayer, M. (2011) Measles vaccination in humanitarian emergencies: a review of recent practice, *Conflict and Health*, 5, 21.

Gupta, R.K., Best, J. and MacMahon, E. (2005) Mumps and the UK epidemic 2005, *British Medical Journal*, 330 (7500): 1132–1135.

Hardt, K., Bonanni, P., King, S., Santos, J.I., El-Hodhod, M., Zimet, G.D. *et al.* (2016) Vaccine strategies: optimising outcomes, *Vaccine*, 34 (52): 6691–6699.

Health and Social Care Information Centre (HSCIC) (2013) *NHS immunisation statistics, England 2012–13*. Available at: http://content.digital.nhs.uk/catalogue/PUB11665/nhs-immu-stat-eng-2012-13-rep.pdf [accessed 9 March 2017].

Helleringer, S., Frimpong, J.A., Abdelwahab, J., Asuming, P., Touré, H., Awoonor-Williams, J. K. *et al.* (2012) Supplementary polio immunization activities and prior use of routine immunization services in non-polio-endemic sub-Saharan Africa, *Bulletin of the World Health Organization*, 90 (7): 495–503.

International Vaccines Access Center (2013) *Vaccines work: India*. Baltimore, MD: Johns Hopkins University. Available at: http://www.jhsph.edu/research/centers-and-institutes/ivac/resources/Impact-of-Vaccines-India.html [accessed 9 March 2017].

Kristensen, D.D., Lorenson, T., Bartholomew, K. and Villadiego, S. (2016) Can thermostable vaccines help address cold-chain challenges? Results from stakeholder interviews in six low- and middle-income countries. *Vaccine*, 34(7): 899–904.

Minor, P.D. (2015) Live attenuated vaccines: historical successes and current challenges, *Virology*, 479/480: 379–392.

Nascimento, I.P. and Leite, L.C.C. (2012) Recombinant vaccines and the development of new vaccine strategies, *Brazilian Journal of Medical and Biological Research*, 45(12): 1102–1111.

NHS Choices (2013) *MMR catch-up campaign targets a million children*, Press release, 25 April. Available at: http://www.nhs.uk/news/2013/04April/Pages/New-MMR-catch-up-campaign-one-million-children-targeted.aspx [accessed 9 March 2017].

NHS Choices (2016) *Meningitis*. Available at: http://www.nhs.uk/Conditions/Meningitis/Pages/Prevention.aspx [accessed 9 March 2017].

Public Health England (PHE) (2015) *Vaccination timeline*. Available at: https://www.gov.uk/government/publications/vaccination-timeline [accessed 9 March 2017].

Shen, A.K., Fields, R. and McQuestion, M. (2014) The future of routine immunization in the developing world: challenges and opportunities, *Global Health: Science and Practice*, 2 (4): 381–394.

Steinglass, R. (2013) Routine immunization: an essential but wobbly platform. *Global Health: Science and Practice*, 1 (3): 295–301.

The Lancet (2010) Retraction – Ileal-lymphoid-nodular hyperplasia, non-specific colitis, and pervasive developmental disorder in children, *Lancet*, 375 (9713): 445.

The Vaccine Confidence Project (2016) *The state of vaccine confidence: 2016*. Available at: http://www.vaccineconfidence.org/research/the-state-of-vaccine-confidence-2016/ [accessed 9 March 2017].

Walkinshaw, E. (2011) Mandatory vaccinations: the international landscape, *Canadian Medical Association Journal*, 183 (16): e1167–e1168.

Weinberg, G.A. and Szilagy, P.G. (2010) Vaccine epidemiology: efficacy, effectiveness, and the translational research roadmap, *Journal of Infectious Diseases*, 201 (11): 1607–1610.

Worboys, M. (2007) Vaccines: conquering untreatable diseases, *British Medical Journal*, 334: s19.

World Health Organization (WHO) (2009) *State of the world's vaccines and immunization*, 3rd edn. Geneva: WHO. Available at: http://apps.who.int/iris/bitstream/10665/44169/1/9789241563864_eng.pdf

World Health Organization (WHO) (2012) *Principles and considerations for adding a vaccine into a national immunization programme: From decision to implementation. Excerpted sections for the April 2012 SAGE session: impact of vaccine introductions on immunization and health systems*. Geneva: WHO. Available at: http://www.who.int/immunization/sage/meetings/2012/april/8_VIGexcerptsYB.pdf

World Health Organization (WHO) (2016a) *Immunization coverage*, Fact sheet, updated September 2016. Available at: http://www.who.int/mediacentre/factsheets/fs378/en/ [accessed 9 March 2017].

World Health Organization (WHO) (2016b) *WHO expanded programme on immunization schedule*. Available at: http://www.who.int/immunization/policy/Immunization_routine_table1.pdf?ua=1 [accessed 10 March 2017].

World Health Organization (WHO) (2016c) *Mission: Yellow fever vaccination*. Available at: http://www.who.int/features/2016/missionvaccination(14).pdf?ua=1 [accessed 9 March 2017].

World Health Organization (WHO) (2017) *Vaccines and diseases*. Available at: http://www.who.int/immunization/diseases/en/ [accessed 9 May 2017].

Yang, J., Acosta, C.J., Si, G., Zeng, J., Li, C., Liang, D. *et al.* (2005) A mass vaccination campaign targeting adults and children to prevent typhoid fever in Hechi. Expanding the use of Vi polysaccharide vaccine in Southeast China: a cluster-randomized trial, *BMC Public Health*, 5 (1): 49.

6

Prevention

Liza Cragg and Will Nutland

Overview

The previous chapter looked at the crucial role immunization plays in preventing communicable disease. This chapter explores the strategies that can be used to prevent outbreaks of communicable disease in addition to immunization, and for those diseases where immunization is not possible. These strategies include reducing exposure and the risk of transmission, reducing the number of contacts infected people have with others, reducing the infectious period and eradicating the disease. The chapter also describes the actions that are commonly used in each of these strategies. The chapter goes on to explain the importance of action to address the causes of communicable disease and support capacity for effective prevention.

Learning objectives

After reading this chapter, you will be able to:

• explain the main strategies for preventing communicable disease
• describe the actions that each of these prevention strategies use
• understand how different strategies are used together to prevent communicable disease
• explain the importance of structural factors, communication, policy-making and healthcare systems in communicable disease prevention

Key terms

Airborne infectious isolation rooms (AIIRs): Single-occupancy patient-care rooms used to isolate people with suspected or confirmed airborne infectious diseases.

Chemoprophylaxis: The practice of taking medications to prevent or reduce the risk of infection, or risk of disease from an infection.

Contract tracing: The process of identifying people who may have come into contact with a person infected with a specific disease.

Healthcare-associated infections (HCAIs):   Infections that occur in patients during the process of care in a hospital or other healthcare facility that were not present or incubating at the time of admission.

Isolation: The process of separating people who have a communicable disease from people who are not infected.

Personal protective equipment (PPE):   Protective clothing or other equipment designed to protect the wearer from injury or infection.

Quarantine: The process of separating and restricting the movement of people who may have been exposed to a contagious disease to see if they develop symptoms.

Social distancing: Voluntary or compulsory measures adopted to prevent people from coming together in ways that might facilitate the spread of a disease.

Strategies to prevent communicable disease

Preventing communicable disease requires breaking the chain of transmission described in Chapter 3. This can be done using different strategies, depending on the characteristics of the communicable disease in question, such as how infectious it is and how it is transmitted. Whichever prevention strategy is used, communication is an essential component of action to prevent communicable disease. This is discussed in more detail in Chapter 8. A widely used and effective strategy to prevent communicable disease is to reduce the number of people who are susceptible by increasing acquired immunity through immunization, as explained in the previous chapter.

Other strategies that can be used to break the chain of transmission include reducing the risk of transmission through actions such as changing how people behave to minimize their risk, good hygiene practices, physical barriers, ventilation, reducing vectors and chemoprophylaxis. Reducing the number of contacts people who are infected with a pathogen have with people who are potentially susceptible is another strategy for prevention. This includes finding cases and tracing the people they have had contact with (known as contact tracing), quarantine and isolation of suspected and confirmed cases, and measures to stop people coming together in ways that might facilitate the spread of the disease (known as social distancing). Another strategy is to reduce the level and/or duration of infectiousness among cases so that they are less likely to infect others. This is primarily achieved by identifying and treating people who are infected. These strategies are discussed in more detail in the following section of this chapter. The relative importance and effectiveness of different strategies will depend on the biological, clinical and epidemiological features of the disease, as well as various contextual factors. Usually, a combination of strategies working together to mutually reinforce each other are required to control communicable disease, rather than one single approach. These strategies need to be planned and implemented in a coordinated way. In some cases, surveillance and prevention can be used to eliminate or eradicate communicable disease.

Reducing the risk of transmission

Health promotion

One way to reduce the risk of transmission of communicable disease is to enable and empower people to change their behaviours through health promotion interventions. Health promotion has been defined as 'the process of enabling people to increase control over, and to improve, their health' (WHO, 1986). It includes increasing people's knowledge and power to avoid or reduce risks. However, it is not limited to addressing specific types of behaviour. Instead, health promotion seeks to generate and emphasize social and personal resources to improve health and wellbeing.

There are a wide range of intervention methods and theories underpinning those methods that are used in health promotion. More in-depth explanation of these can be found in *Health Promotion Practice* (Nutland and Cragg, 2015) and *Health Promotion Theory* (Cragg *et al.*, 2013), both of which are part of the Understanding Public Health series. Some health promotion interventions are aimed at preventing the transmission of a specific communicable disease. One example is the mass media campaign to educate people about how to reduce the risk of catching influenza, as illustrated in Figure 6.1. Other interventions focus on actions to reduce the risk of infection from a number of potential infectious agents.

Research has shown that interventions on behaviour change can play an important role in preventing communicable disease. However, how effective these interventions are will depend on the context and the characteristics of the disease (Verelst *et al.*, 2016). It is also important to recognize that behaviour change should not be seen as the only preventative strategy required. Behaviour needs to be understood in the context of underlying socio-cultural, economic, political and legal factors. For example, HIV prevention programmes in sub-Saharan Africa initially focused on preventing the sexual transmission of HIV through the ABC message, 'Abstinence, Be faithful, Use a Condom'. However, by the mid-2000s it became clear that this approach was not effective. HIV prevention now recognizes the need to take into account underlying socio-cultural, economic, political, legal and other contextual factors and uses a combination of biomedical, behavioural and structural interventions (UNAIDS, 2010). Importantly, if individuals do not adjust their behaviours in ways an intervention anticipates, those individuals should not be blamed or stigmatized. Blame and stigmatization can result in individuals being unable or unwilling to seek treatment and support, which can actually increase the rate of infection.

CATCH IT
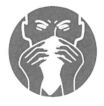

Germs spread easily. Always carry tissues and use them to catch your cough or sneeze.

BIN IT
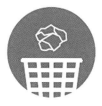

Germs can live for several hours on tissues. Dispose of your tissue as soon as possible.

KILL IT
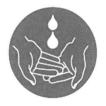

Hands can transfer germs to every surface you touch. Clean your hands as soon as you can.

Figure 6.1 NHS advertisement in the UK, during the H1N1 pandemic

Source: https://www.england.nhs.uk/south/wp-content/uploads/sites/6/2017/09/catch-bin-kill.pdf

Hygiene

Hygiene refers to behaviours that improve cleanliness and promote good health, including frequent hand washing, face washing, teeth cleaning and body washing. Hand washing is one the most effective measures that people can take to avoid becoming ill and spreading infectious agents to others. As explained in Chapter 3, infectious agents can get onto people's hands when they use the toilet, when they handle objects that have been contaminated by other people sneezing, coughing or touching them, or when they touch food that is contaminated. When these infectious agents get onto a person's hands, they can enter the body through, for example, the mouth, nose or eyes. They can also be passed on to another person or contaminate food or drinks.

Effective hand washing has been shown to substantially reduce the risk of infectious disease, particularly respiratory and diarrhoeal infections (Aiello *et al.*, 2008). Educating people about this and explaining effective hand-washing technique is a frequent health promotion intervention used in communicable disease control. It is also key to infection control in healthcare facilities, as discussed later in this chapter. Effective hand washing requires five steps (CDC, 2015):

1. Wetting the hands with clean, running water (warm or cold) and applying soap.
2. Lathering the hands by rubbing them together with the soap, including the backs of the hands, between the fingers, and under the nails.
3. Scrubbing the hands for at least 20 seconds.
4. Rinsing hands well under clean, running water.
5. Drying the hands using a clean towel or air drying them.

If soap and water are not available, an alcohol-based hand sanitizer that contains at least 60% alcohol can be used. It is especially important to wash hands at key points, including: before, during and after preparing food; before eating food; before and after caring for someone who is sick; before and after treating a cut or wound; after using the toilet; after blowing your nose, coughing or sneezing; and after touching an animal, animal feed, or animal waste or rubbish.

Physical barriers

Physical barriers include any item that can consistently and effectively prevent an infectious agent travelling from the portal of exit in the original host to the portal of entry of the susceptible individual. Many physical barriers are items worn on or around the body, which may be designed to protect the wearer and/or people the wearer comes into contact with from infection. Some physical barriers are especially designed to be worn in certain high-risk situations, including personal protective equipment (PPE). However, some are for more general use, such as long-sleeved clothing to protect against mosquito bites. The most common physical barriers used to prevent communicable disease are described below.

Sexual barriers

Sexual barriers include male condoms, female condoms and dental dams. If used correctly, sexual barriers can reduce the risk of sexually transmitted infections including HIV. They can also provide protection against other diseases that may be transmitted through sexual intercourse, like Zika and Ebola virus disease (EVD). However, they do not eliminate all risk, especially if they are not used correctly.

Facemasks

A facemask is a loose-fitting, disposable item that creates a physical barrier between the mouth and nose of the wearer and potential contaminants in the immediate environment. Facemasks are usually used in healthcare settings, for example surgical or dental masks. They may come with or without a face shield. If worn properly, a facemask helps block large-particle droplets, splashes, sprays or splatter that may contain infectious agents from reaching the mouth and nose. Facemasks also help reduce the exposure of other people to the wearer's saliva and respiratory secretions.

Gloves

Protective latex or vinyl gloves are frequently worn by healthcare providers during health care for two reasons: first, to protect hands from contamination with organic matter and microorganisms; and second, to reduce the risks of transmission of microorganisms to both patients and staff. Gloves should be worn for invasive procedures, contact with sterile sites and non-intact skin or mucous membranes, and all activities that have been assessed as carrying a risk of exposure to blood, body fluids, secretions or excretions, or to sharp or contaminated instruments. However, while the use of gloves as a method of barrier protection reduces the risk of contamination, it does not eliminate this risk. Gloves may become damaged and hands may become contaminated during the removal of gloves. Gloves must only be used once and cannot be washed. They must be put on immediately before the medical act and removed as soon as the activity is completed (NICE, 2012).

Aprons and gowns

Aprons and gowns are used as PPE over clothes to avoid clothes becoming contaminated with infectious material. Healthcare workers are advised that when delivering direct patient care, they should wear a disposable plastic apron if there is a risk that clothing may be exposed to blood, body fluids, secretions or excretions, or to wear a long-sleeved fluid-repellent gown if there is a risk of extensive splashing of these body fluids onto skin or clothing (NICE, 2012).

Hazardous material suits

A hazardous material suit, or HAZMAT suit, is an impermeable whole-body garment used by healthcare workers when there is a significant risk posed by the infectious agent with which the patients they are treating are infected. They are used, for example, by healthcare staff treating EVD. There are different types of HAZMAT suit offering varying degrees of protection. They can be very uncomfortable to wear and staff need training in how to use them. They also may need help to put them on and take them off safely.

Respirators

A respirator is a personal protective device worn on the face that covers the nose and mouth, and sometimes the whole face. It reduces the wearer's risk of inhaling hazardous airborne particles, including infectious agents. Respirators are used as medical and occupational health devices. They must be individually fitted to be effective.

Eye protection

Infectious agents can also enter the body through the eyes. Protective eyewear offers protection against physical splashing of infected substances into the eyes when used properly. Expert opinion recommends that face and eye protection be worn where there is a risk of blood, body fluids, secretions or excretions splashing into the face and eyes (NICE, 2012).

Bed nets

Bed nets are also a type of physical barrier used to prevent insect bites when people are sleeping and so can prevent certain vector-borne diseases. This method of prevention is discussed in more detail below as part of vector control measures.

Ventilation

There is sufficient evidence to demonstrate the association between ventilation, air movements in buildings and the transmission of infectious diseases such as measles, tuberculosis (TB), chickenpox, influenza, smallpox and SARS (Li *et al.*, 2007). The WHO guidelines on 'Natural Ventilation for Infection Control in Health-Care Settings' recommend that to help prevent airborne infections, adequate ventilation is necessary in all patient-care areas in healthcare facilities. When natural ventilation alone cannot satisfy the recommended ventilation requirements, alternative ventilation systems should be considered. If that is not adequate, mechanical ventilation should be used (WHO, 2009).

Technologically advanced healthcare facilities such as large hospitals in high-income counties may use airborne infectious isolation rooms (AIIRs), sometimes called negative pressure rooms. These are single-occupancy patient-care rooms used to isolate people with suspected or confirmed airborne infectious diseases. Environmental factors are controlled in AIIRs to minimize the transmission of infectious agents.

Eliminating reservoirs and vector control

Another way to reduce the risk of transmission is to reduce or eliminate the reservoir of a disease. Where the reservoir is an infected person, this is usually done by medically treating the person so as to eliminate or reduce the infectious agent within the host, thereby reducing the duration of the infectious period and/or the probability of transmitting the disease during the infectious period. This is discussed in more detail below. If the reservoir is an animal, measures can be taken to eliminate the infectious agent from the affected animals to prevent them infecting humans. Measures include: animal vaccination; treatment of infected animals; flea and tick control; requirements to notify authorities of diseased animals; controls on the movement of animals; rigid infection control in facilities that handle animals routinely such as laboratories and farms; and public education on safe practices such as avoiding close contact with animals so as not to be scratched or bitten. Where these measures are not feasible or effective, government authorities may also organize animal culls. However, animal culls are controversial and may not be effective. For example, dogs are the source of the vast majority of human rabies deaths, contributing up to 99% of all rabies transmissions to humans. The WHO recommends vaccinating dogs as a cost-effective strategy for preventing rabies in people, as vaccinating at least 70% of dogs, including strays, can break the transmission pathway. Dog vaccination reduces deaths attributable to rabies and the need for post-exposure prophylaxis (PEP), a form of treatment given after a person has been bitten or scratched to reduce the risk of them developing rabies. However, governments in some countries continue to endorse culls of stray dogs to control the spread of rabies, although there is no evidence that removal of dogs alone has an impact on the incidence of rabies (WHO, 2004).

For vector-borne diseases, controlling vectors can be an effective preventative strategy. Mosquitoes are the most well-known disease vector. Other vectors include ticks, flies, sandflies, fleas, triatomine bugs and some freshwater aquatic snails. Controlling these vectors is not always easy to achieve, as vectors often reside in large or difficult to access environments, such as bodies of water or on wild animals. The short life cycles of vectors, along with other features related to their natural histories, can also make them resilient to efforts aimed at reducing their population densities.

Controlling vectors involves public education to explain to people how to protect themselves, for example by eliminating pools of stagnant water where possible, and using bed nets. Another way of controlling vectors involves the use of chemicals to kill the vectors and their larvae through fogging or spraying. Challenges associated with chemical controls include: the potential for adverse effects in people and ecosystems exposed to the chemicals; the acceptability of this method to local communities; the human resources and other costs required; and increasing resistance among vectors in some areas to the chemicals commonly used. Strategies for vector control need to be adapted to local conditions and to take account of epidemiological data on the incidence of diseases and at-risk populations, and entomological data on the vectors including insecticide resistance and vector behaviour.

For vector control to prevent malaria, the WHO recommends two core, broadly applicable interventions: ensuring that all people living in areas where the risk of malaria is high are protected through the provision, use and timely replacement of long-lasting insecticide-treated nets (LLINs); and, where appropriate, the application of indoor residual spraying, which involves coating the walls and other surfaces of a house with a residual insecticide. Supplementary methods may be appropriate in specific settings, for instance larval source management where mosquitoes' aquatic habitats are few, fixed and findable. Because of growing evidence of physiological resistance of mosquitoes to insecticides, the WHO stresses that it is crucial to closely plan, implement and monitor vector control programmes (WHO, 2015a).

Research is ongoing into new approaches to control vectors, including genetically modifying mosquitoes so that they become resistant to the infectious agents they spread. As these approaches are species-specific and not dependent on insecticides, they present opportunities for more targeted and environmentally friendly strategies (Yakob and Walker, 2017). One such initiative to modify mosquitoes has shown early promise in blocking the transmission of dengue fever (Walker *et al.*, 2011).

Chemoprophylaxis

Chemoprophylaxis refers to the practice of taking medications to prevent or reduce the risk of infection, or of developing disease from an infection. Chemoprophylaxis is different from immunization in that it does not lead to the development of acquired immunity to an infectious agent. Instead, it stops the infectious agent causing disease in the person taking chemoprophylaxis. It only works while the person is taking the chemoprophylactic. The medication, dosing and duration of chemoprophylaxis required depends on the characteristics of the specific infectious agent and the needs of the individual. Some forms of chemoprophylaxis are taken before and during a period of increased exposure to a risk (known as pre-exposure prophylaxis).

For example, chemoprophylaxis for malaria is often taken during a period when travelling in a malaria endemic country. Others forms of chemoprophylaxis are taken after risk exposure (PEP), for example post-exposure vaccination to prevent rabies in a person who has been bitten by an animal who may be infected.

Chemoprophylaxis can be very effective at preventing the development of disease and limiting the severity of disease in individuals who take it. By reducing the number of people infected, and/or by reducing the infectiousness of those who become infected, it also contributes to reducing the human reservoir of an infectious agent. However, it has its disadvantages and limitations. These include: the potential for side-effects of the medications used and/or interactions with other medications; the risk of the infectious agent developing resistance to the drugs used in chemoprophylaxis; the need for strict adherence to maximize effectiveness; the costs of chemoprophylaxis medications; and the need for medical supervision. For these reasons, chemoprophylaxis is in general not used for extended periods or for whole populations. However, chemoprophylaxis can be very useful for groups and individuals who experience a particularly high risk of a disease and for short-term use. Some common examples of chemoprophylaxis are described below.

Malaria chemoprophylaxis

Chemoprophylaxis is often used to prevent malaria in travellers to areas where malaria is prevalent. Several different drugs can be used, including atovaquone/proguanil, chloroquine, doxycycline and mefloquine. None of these give total protection, and antimalarial drug resistance is a major challenge to malaria control. Chemoprophylaxis therefore needs to be combined with the use of personal protective measures such as insect repellent, long sleeves, long pants, and sleeping in a mosquito-free setting or using an insecticide-treated bed net.

Perioperative antibiotic prophylaxis

Perioperative antibiotic prophylaxis is the use of antibiotics to prevent bacterial infections in patients who have had surgery. While effective in preventing infections, research shows perioperative antibiotic prophylaxis is associated with increases in antibiotic resistance and healthcare costs and that it is often used without a good reason (Zweigner *et al.*, 2013). Therefore, guidelines now recommend that antibiotic prophylaxis is not routinely used for clean, uncomplicated surgery and is reserved for certain, more risky types of surgery (NICE, 2017).

HIV pre-exposure prophylaxis

Pre-exposure prophylaxis, or PrEP, is used to protect people who are HIV negative but who have an increased risk of HIV infection. The medications currently used are tenofovir and emtricitabine in combination. When someone is exposed to HIV, the medications stop the virus from establishing a permanent infection. When taken consistently, PrFP has been shown to almost totally reduce the risk of HIV infection. However, PrEP is much less effective if it is not taken consistently (CDC, 2016).

HIV PEP

PEP means taking medication after being potentially exposed to reduce the likelihood of being infected with HIV. People can be accidentally exposed to HIV through healthcare work or through unprotected sex or sexual assault. PEP uses a 28-day course of antiretrovirals (ARVs), which have been used to prevent infection in case of accidental exposures for many years. PEP should be initiated as early as possible and ideally within 72 hours. If started soon after exposure, PEP can reduce the risk of HIV infection by over 80% (WHO, 2014).

Rabies PEP

In countries or areas at risk of rabies, a person who has received an animal bite, scratch or other contact with an animal suspected to be rabid might require PEP. This involves active immunization through administration of the rabies vaccine in a multi-dose regimen over several weeks. This may also be combined with 'passive immunization', involving intravenous administration of immunoglobulin (antibodies) against the rabies virus, if the type of exposure is deemed to be high risk. Immediate wound cleansing with soap and water after contact with a suspected rabid animal is also essential. Strict adherence to WHO-recommended guidelines for optimal post-exposure rabies prophylaxis virtually guarantees protection from the disease (WHO, 2004).

Reducing the contacts of people infected

Contact tracing

Contract tracing is the process of identifying people who may have come into contact with a person infected with a specific disease. Contact tracing is undertaken as part of communicable disease surveillance, as discussed in Chapter 4. It also is an important mechanism for preventing the transmission of communicable disease, as it identifies people who may have been infected but who do not yet have symptoms. This then allows them to be treated or isolated before they can go on to infect others. For sexually transmitted diseases, contact tracing is generally limited to sexual partners. Because contact tracing is time-consuming and resource-intensive, it is usually used only for potentially serious diseases with a relatively low prevalence, such as TB and HIV. For some diseases, contact

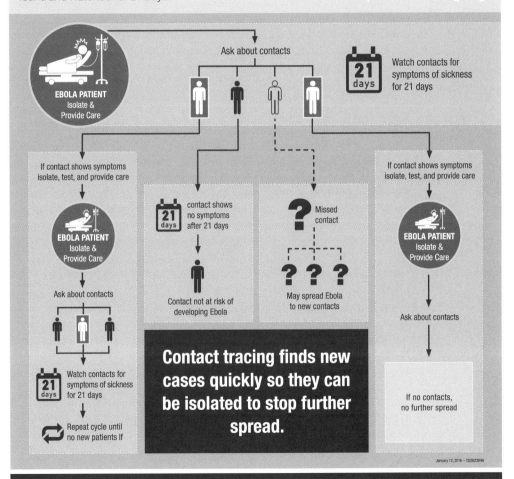

Figure 6.2 Infographic on contact tracing for Ebola virus disease produced by the Disease Control and Prevention (CDC)

Source: CDC, https://www.cdc.gov/vhf/ebola/pdf/contact-tracing.pdf.

tracing is an important tool in stopping the spread of an epidemic; for example, contact tracing was used extensively during the outbreak of EVD in West Africa in 2014. The infographic in Figure 6.2 shows how contact tracing was used in this case. Research indicates that several factors are important if contact tracing is to be effective. These include: the period of individual infectivity, the variability in time between infection and symptom-based detection, and the efficiency and speed of the tracing process (Klinkenberg *et al.*, 2006).

Isolation and quarantine

Isolation is the process of separating people who have a communicable disease from uninfected and potentially susceptible people. Isolation is generally used in hospital facilities to separate a patient with a communicable disease from other patients. A special isolation room that is occupied by a single patient is usually used. Larger isolation facilities are used during outbreaks of highly infectious diseases such as EVD. Isolation is also sometimes used to protect patients who are very immunosuppressed from circulating infectious agents.

Quarantine refers to the process of separating and restricting the movement of people who were (or may have been) exposed to a contagious disease to see if they become sick. As was explained in Chapter 1, quarantine was widely used throughout the world from the medieval period until the early twentieth century. Although it is not widely used now, most national governments retain legal powers to bring in quarantine provisions. Governments may also use quarantine as part of border control systems. In the USA, for example, quarantine stations are located at ports of entry and land–border crossings where international travellers arrive. They are staffed with quarantine medical and public health officers from the CDC who decide whether people who are ill can enter the USA and what measures should be taken to prevent the spread of infectious diseases (CDC, 2014).

Quarantine has the potential to create fear and stigma, which can prevent people seeking treatment and actually increase infections. Research has suggested that while isolation of confirmed cases is a desirable public health measure, quarantine can result in significant social, psychological and economic costs. In addition, the number of additional infections that can be averted through the use of quarantine, provided isolation is used effectively, is very small (Day *et al.*, 2006).

Social distancing

Social distancing is a term used to describe actions to stop or slow down the spread of a highly contagious disease through reducing contact rates among the population at risk. It can include actions that people take voluntarily and spontaneously to limit their contact with others after hearing about a disease threat, such as working from home or avoiding public transport. It can also include actions taken by public health or other government authorities to limit large groups of people coming together, for example closing schools, cancelling mass gathering events and suspending mass transport systems. Social distancing causes social, economic and other forms of disruption and may cause significant anxiety. Therefore, it may not be considered acceptable by populations and governments. There is limited evidence about the effectiveness of social distancing. One mathematical modelling study concluded that to be effective it requires reducing contacts drastically in the earliest stages of an outbreak, thereby suppressing the epidemic quickly (Maharaj and Kleczkowski, 2012).

 Activity 6.1

Read the case study of norovirus below and reflect on the questions that follow it.

In January 2014, a large cruise ship, carrying over 3000 passengers and 1000 crew members, set forth on a leisure cruise. During the excursion, a number of passengers and crew started to display symptoms of vomiting and diarrhoea. The case count escalated leading to 634 passengers (20.6% of the passengers) and 55 crew members (4.7% of the crew) becoming infected. The pathogen was subsequently confirmed to be norovirus. Noroviruses thrive in areas where people live, work or interact in close quarters, such as cruise ships or institutional facilities. People usually become infected by eating food or drinking liquids that are contaminated with norovirus or by touching surfaces or objects contaminated with norovirus and then putting their fingers in their mouth. Infection can also occur by having contact with someone who is infected with norovirus, including caring for or sharing food or eating utensils with someone with norovirus illness. Although highly contagious, norovirus usually causes only mild-to-moderate, self-limiting disease, with symptoms lasting around 12–60 hours. Cases are most infectious when symptomatic and during the 2–3 days following recovery. Noroviruses are very stable in the environment, relatively resistant to disinfectant, and can survive temperatures as high as 140°F, including quick steaming processes that are often used for cooking shellfish.

1. If you were in charge of the response to the outbreak described above, what would your education programme for passengers consist

of? Would your information to crew members be any different (how and why)?

2. Given that cruise ships are often subject to outbreaks of norovirus, what specific measures might you enact to prevent outbreaks in the future?

3. What other measure would you take?

Feedback

- You should make passengers aware of the outbreak and encourage them to report if they become sick, with clear instructions on who should report (that is, anyone with vomiting or diarrhoea) and how (for example, by providing a 24-hour medical helpline number). You should explain to them that it is very important that they practise good hand hygiene (as outlined above), and maybe recommend that sick passengers remain in their cabins until 48 hours after symptoms subside (cabin service could be provided). You should explain that they should not prepare food or look after other people if they are sick. In addition, you should explain to all staff that fruit and vegetables need to be washed properly and seafood needs to be cooked thoroughly. As with the passengers, you should explain to staff that if they are sick they must report it immediately, that they must not prepare any food or care for anyone until at least 48 hours after their symptoms subside. You should explain that soiled fabrics must be properly cleaned at high temperatures.

- The WHO reports that to prevent or reduce outbreaks of gastroenteritis caused by norovirus, ships should follow enhanced food and water sanitation measures. Surfaces should be disinfected and hand gel dispensers provided at strategic locations throughout the ship and passengers and crew urged to use them. Some cruise companies ask that those who present with gastrointestinal symptoms at on-board medical centres be put into isolation until at least 24 hours after their last symptoms, and some ships also isolate asymptomatic contacts for 24 hours (WHO, 2017). Cruise ships are required to investigate, record and report cases of passengers and crew members that say they have symptoms of illness to the relevant port authorities.

- There is no specific medicine to treat people with norovirus illness. However, it is very important they drink plenty of liquids to replace fluid lost from vomiting and diarrhoea. This will help prevent dehydration. Dehydration can lead to serious problems. It is important to make sure vulnerable people, such as people living with chronic disease, older people and young children, do not become dehydrated.

Reducing the duration and level of infectiousness among cases

Effective health care can reduce mortality and morbidity from communicable disease. However, it is also plays a crucial role in reducing transmission and preventing infections. As discussed in Chapters 2 and 3, this is because communicable disease spreads as infectious agents are transmitted from person to person. Providing effective medical treatment to someone who is infected can reduce the period during which they are infected and, therefore, the period during which they can transmit the disease to other people. For example, based on the simple principle of people being non-infectious after they are cured, research indicates that the expansion of direct-acting antivirals could decrease population transmission of hepatitis C virus (Hagan et al., 2013). Even where treatment does not lead to a cure, it can contribute to reducing the infectious period and/or the level of infectiousness among cases. For example, a landmark study in 2011 demonstrated that early initiation of antiretroviral therapy (ART) reduced rates of sexual transmission of HIV-1 (Cohen et al., 2011). More recent research has demonstrated that high rates of ART treatment coverage in a community can result in substantial population-level reductions in the rate of new HIV infections in sub-Saharan Africa (Tanser et al., 2013).

Policies and practices that encourage the early detection and treatment of diseases should be a routine part of health care. This requires funding for diagnosis and treatment services, policies and practices designed to prevent infections and adverse events related to healthcare, data management and sharing policies that optimize secure exchange of health information and advance public health goals, occupational safety policies and practices that protect both patients and healthcare workers (for example, improving influenza vaccination rates among hospital personnel) (CDC, 2011). The roles that different parts of the health systems play in this are discussed in more detail in Chapter 10.

Disease eradication and elimination

The most effective and permanent way of preventing a communicable disease is to eradicate it. Disease eradication is defined as the permanent reduction to zero of the worldwide incidence of infection. Eradication requires close surveillance and highly effective preventative strategies, such as an effective vaccine, specially designed for the features of the specific disease. Chapter 1 addressed the key points in the successful campaign to eradicate smallpox and highlighted that activities to complete the eradication of polio are now under way. A campaign to eradicate Guinea worm disease is also under way and cases have been reduced from an estimated 3.5 million in 1986 to 25 in 2016, which were restricted to just three countries (The Carter Center, 2017).

However, disease eradication is difficult and costly to achieve. In addition, it is only feasible when a number of conditions are in place, including biological and epidemiological feasibility, adequate public health infrastructure, sufficient funding, and sustained political and societal will. Biological feasibility requires that an effective intervention is available to interrupt transmission of the agent there are available practical diagnostic tools with sufficient sensitivity and specificity to detect levels of infection that can lead to transmission, and humans are essential for the life cycle of the agent, which has no other vertebrate reservoir and does not amplify in the environment (Dowdle and Cochi, 2011). The WHO is the only organization that can officially certify the eradication of a disease.

Where eradication of a disease is not feasible, it may be possible to eliminate it. Elimination is defined as the reduction to zero of the incidence of a specified disease in a defined geographical area as a result of deliberate efforts, and continued intervention measures are required. Many vaccine-preventable diseases, including rubella, diphtheria and measles, have been eliminated in high- and middle-income countries. Strategies and resolutions are also in place to eliminate malaria and certain neglected tropical diseases, including lymphatic filariasis and onchocerciasis (river blindness). However, it is important to stress that where a disease has been eliminated, there is still a need for continued surveillance and prevention to ensure that the infectious agent does not re-emerge and establish sustained transmission again.

Integrating communicable disease prevention

The strategies described above need to be integrated into broader policies that address the causes of communicable disease and support capacity for effective prevention. These include evidence-based policies, structural interventions, overall strengthening of healthcare and public health systems, and preventing HCAI. As Chapter 4 highlighted, surveillance is also central to the prevention of communicable diseases.

Evidence-based policies

Communicable disease prevention requires consistent and coherent policies that cover the wide range of sectors involved, including health care, food safety and standards, housing, sanitation, animal management, environmental control and other social determinants of health. Policies need to be based on the best available evidence of what is effective in a particular context. This means policy-makers require hard evidence to inform their decision-making. In practice, the available evidence may be limited or of poor quality. Decision-makers may also have a short time in which to consider the available evidence and make decisions, particularly if there is an outbreak. Therefore, evidence-based decision-making for communicable disease control requires integrating the best available evidence with the knowledge and considered judgements from stakeholders and experts to benefit the needs of a population (ECDC, 2011). Policy development needs to extend beyond the public health and healthcare communities to engage stakeholders in other sectors and members of the public, including at-risk and vulnerable groups.

In addition to coherent policies that are based on the best evidence, communicable disease prevention requires adequate infrastructure, financing, staff and other resources to put these policies into practice. Resources need to be distributed geographically so as to be accessible to and meet the needs of the whole population. Local, regional and national levels of government need to be properly coordinated and linked with relevant international guidance. Government agencies need to coordinate with non-governmental organizations (NGOs), businesses, community leaders and the public, as these all have an important role to play in communicable disease prevention.

Structural interventions

The social determinants of health and their influence on communicable disease were described in Chapter 2. People in low-income countries are more likely to have inadequate food, unclean water, poor sanitation, overcrowded and poor housing, lack of medical care and other services, and poor environments. This means they are more likely to be exposed to infectious agents, are less able to resist infections and have poor access to preventative and curative health care. Consequently, they have much higher rates of mortality and morbidity from communicable diseases. For example, the WHO data from 2015 indicates the under-5 mortality rate in low-income countries was 76 deaths per 1000 live births – about 11 times the average rate in high-income countries, and the majority of these deaths are a result of communicable disease (WHO, 2015b). However, even within high-income countries, the level and distribution of wealth within a society plays a significant role in determining vulnerabilities to communicable diseases. For example, TB prevalence rates show significant associations with wealth inequality in European Union (EU) member states (Semenza et al., 2010).

Strategies to prevent communicable disease, which do not address the underlying factors that cause some population groups to be more at risk than others, are unlikely to be effective. For example, a behaviour change campaign that seeks to improve hand washing and food hygiene is not likely to be successful in a community that does not have access to adequate clean water. Therefore, structural interventions that address the social determinants of health and health inequities between countries, and within countries, need to be considered as part of action to prevent communicable diseases. These interventions include provision of health services, education, housing, sanitation, employment, transport and quality environments. Many of these actions are outside the remit of health systems and so require coordinated action across sectors by national governments, the WHO, United Nations (UN) agencies and civil society organizations.

Healthcare and public health systems

Healthcare and public health systems are essential to communicable disease prevention. Chapter 4 looked at the role of healthcare and public health systems in communicable disease surveillance. That chapter explained the role of public health preventative strategies including behaviour change to reduce the risk of transmission. It also explained how appropriate and prompt health care can prevent communicable disease by reducing the infectious period. Healthcare and public health systems also play a key role in other prevention strategies, including chemoprophylaxis, vector control and isolation. To fulfil these essential roles, healthcare and public health systems require adequate financing, information systems, sufficient physical infrastructure, appropriate and ongoing training of staff, performance management systems, and leadership and governance. Healthcare and public health systems should also focus on patients' needs. In Chapter 10, we explain more about how health systems are structured and their role in communicable disease control.

 Activity 6.2

Read the case study of rabies below and reflect on the questions that follow it.

Rabies is a viral disease that is almost always fatal following the onset of clinical signs. It is estimated to kill more than 50,000 people every year. Up to 99% of human cases are caused by zoonotic transmission of the virus from domestic dogs. Rabies is present on all continents with the exception of Antarctica, but more than 95% of human deaths occur in Asia and Africa. Around 40% of those affected are under the age of 15.

1. What do you think are the best ways of preventing the transmission of rabies?
2. What social determinants of health might impact on the transmission of rabies?

Feedback

1. Prevention strategies you could have suggested include: public education on the need to avoid stray dogs; responsible dog ownerhip;

the importance of immediate thorough wound cleansing; the need to seek immediate medical help and the importance of having pet dogs vaccinated; teaching children how to avoid animal bites; making treatment available, including wound cleaning and PEP against rabies; vaccination of people in endemic areas; mass vaccination programmes for all dogs including stray dogs; offering free dog vaccination and registration to owners as an incentive to pay particular attention to their pets. You may also have included the importance of good data and the need for funding, healthcare infrastructure and leadership.

2. More than 95% of human deaths occur in Asia and Africa. Deaths are frequently not reported, so surveillance is difficult. Rabies is a neglected disease of poor and vulnerable populations. Many victims live in remote rural communities where access to health care is poor and human vaccines and PEP are not readily available or accessible. The average cost of rabies post-exposure prophylaxis is around US$40 in Africa and US$49 in Asia, where the average daily income is about US$1–2 per person in poor populations. For such populations, access to basic healthcare services and health insurance coverage is often limited. Therefore, often those affected cannot access or afford appropriate treatment. Governments in low-income countries are forced to prioritize activities, based on the leading causes of morbidity and mortality. Rabies, although it affects many people globally and is completely preventable and fatal, is not a leading cause of mortality and so may not be addressed effectively. More information on control and elimination strategies for rabies can be found on the WHO website at: http://www.who.int/rabies/control/en/.

Preventing healthcare-associated infections

Healthcare-associated infections (HCAIs) are infections that occur in patients during the process of care in a hospital or other healthcare facility that were not present or incubating at the time of admission. HCAIs can affect patients in any type of setting where they receive care. Signs and symptoms of HCAIs can also present after discharge. HCAIs are sometimes referred to as nosocomial or hospital-acquired infections. They are the most frequent adverse events in healthcare delivery globally. Hundreds of millions of patients are affected worldwide each year, resulting in significant mortality, suffering, prolonged hospital stay and financial losses. A systematic review by the WHO found prevalence of HCAIs in high-income countries of around 7%, meaning for every 100 patients around seven have a HCAI. In low- and middle-income countries, fewer data are available but prevalence of HCAIs is estimated to be around 10% to 15% (WHO, 2011).

Infection prevention and control is the term used to describe action to prevent HCAIs.

Many healthcare systems produce guidelines in infection prevention and control for health facilities. Guidelines for England, for example, are produced and updated regularly based on the best available evidence. The latest guidelines include specific recommendations and standards around five themes: cleaning standards for facilities and equipment; effective hand washing and hand decontamination for staff, patients and visitors; correct use of personal protective equipment; safe use and disposal of injection needles; and procedures for invasive devices, sterile fluids and medication, surgical incisions and wound care (Loveday *et al.*, 2014). Figure 6.3 gives an example of an education poster for healthcare staff on hand hygiene. Other important measures include immunization of staff, appropriate antibiotic usage policies, and minimizing patient length of stay where possible. A dedicated infection control team for surveillance and control at each health facility is essential. Measures to improve awareness and accountability of staff, for example through producing surgeon-specific HCAI rates and through audits of wards and theatres, can also be beneficial (Noah, 2006).

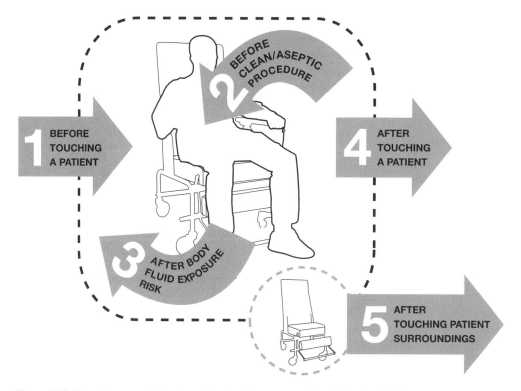

Figure 6.3 'Your 5 moments for hand hygiene' poster produced by the WHO as part of an education campaign for healthcare workers

Source: WHO, http://www.who.int/gpsc/5may/tools/workplace_reminders/Your_5_Moments_For_Hand_Hygiene_Poster_Chair.pdf

---

✏️ **Activity 6.3**

Go back to the list of you made for Activity 2.1 in Chapter 2 of the different communicable diseases that you have been affected by. Based on your reading so far, is there anything you or anyone else could have done to prevent their transmission? Can you think of the reasons why this action wasn't taken at the time?

Feedback

Your response will depend on the diseases you identified. For example, you might have reflected that one of the diseases you had as a child is now vaccine-preventable but the vaccine wasn't available at the time. You might have concluded that the many cold viruses you have had may potentially have been prevented by better hand hygiene. You might have been affected by a gastrointestinal infection that could have been prevented by improved food safety.

Summary

This chapter has explained the strategies that can be used to break the chain of transmission in order to prevent communicable disease. These strategies include reducing the risk of transmission, reducing the number of contacts an infectious person has and reducing the infectious period. Rather than one approach, several different strategies are usually required. Whatever strategies are used, they will generally need to be underpinned by actions to address the social determinants of health that contribute to communicable disease. They also require healthcare and public health infrastructure and evidence-based policies. Maintaining a patient focus and engaging all stakeholders is also essential. Together with surveillance and immunization, these preventative strategies are used to control communicable disease. The next chapter explores how control measures need to be adapted and applied in an outbreak situation.

References

Aiello, A.E., Coulborn, R.M., Perez, V. and Larson, E.L. (2008) Effect of hand hygiene on infectious disease risk in the community setting: a meta-analysis, *American Journal of Public Health*, 98 (8): 1372–1381.

Centers for Disease Control and Prevention (CDC) (2011) *A CDC framework for preventing infectious diseases: Sustaining the essentials and innovating for the future*. Atlanta, GA: CDC.

Centers for Disease Control and Prevention (CDC) (2014) *Quarantine and isolation*. Available at: https://www.cdc.gov/quarantine/quarantinestations.html [accessed 5 March 2017].

Centers for Disease Control and Prevention (CDC) (2015) *Handwashing: Clean hands save lives*. Available at: https://www.cdc.gov/handwashing/when-how-handwashing.html [accessed 5 March 2017].

Centers for Disease Control and Prevention (CDC) (2016) *Pre-exposure prophylaxis (PrEP)*. Available at: https://www.cdc.gov/hiv/risk/prep/ [accessed 5 March 2017].

Cohen, M.S., Chen, Y.Q., McCauley, M., Gamble, T., Hosseinipour, M.C., Kumarasamy, N. *et al.* (2011) Prevention of HIV-1 infection with early antiretroviral therapy, *New England Journal of Medicine*, 365 (6): 493–505.

Cragg, L., Davies, M. and Macdowall, W. (eds.) (2013) *Health Promotion Theory*, 2nd edn. Maidenhead: Open University Press.

Day, T., Park, A., Madras, N., Gumel, A. and Wu, J. (2006) When is quarantine a useful control strategy for emerging infectious diseases?, *American Journal of Epidemiology*, 163 (5): 479–485.

Dowdle, W.R. and Cochi, S.L. (2011) The principles and feasibility of disease eradication, *Vaccine*, 29 (suppl. 4): D70–D73.

European Centre for Disease Prevention and Control (ECDC) (2011) *Evidence-based methodologies for public health: How to assess the best available evidence when time is limited and there is lack of sound evidence*. Stockholm: ECDC.

Hagan, L.M., Wolpe, P.R. and Schinazi, R.F. (2013) Treatment as prevention and cure towards global eradication of hepatitis C virus, *Trends in Microbiology*, 21 (12): 625–633.

Klinkenberg, D., Fraser, C. and Heesterbeek, H. (2006) The effectiveness of contact tracing in emerging epidemics, *PLoS ONE*, 1 (1): e12.

Li, Y., Leung, G.M., Tang, J.W., Yang, X., Chao, C.Y.H., Lin, J.Z. *et al.* (2007) Role of ventilation in airborne transmission of infectious agents in the built environment – a multidisciplinary systematic review, *Indoor Air*, 17: 2–18.

Loveday, H.P., Wilson, J.A., Pratt, R.J., Golsorkhi, M., Tingle, A., Bak, A. *et al.* (2014) epic3: National evidence-based guidelines for preventing healthcare-associated infections in NHS hospitals in England, *Journal of Hospital Infection*, 86: S1–S70.

Maharaj, S. and Kleczkowski, A. (2012) Controlling epidemic spread by social distancing: do it well or not at all, *BMC Public Health*, 12: 679.

National Institute for Health and Care Excellence (NICE) (2012) 7. Standard principles for the use of personal protective equipment, in *Infection: prevention and control of healthcare-associated infections in primary and community care – Partial update of NICE Clinical Guideline 2*, NICE Clinical Guideline No. 139. London: Royal College of Physicians. Available at: https://www.ncbi.nlm.nih.gov/books/NBK115274/.

National Institute for Health and Care Excellence (NICE) (2017) *Surgical site infections: prevention and treatment*, Clinical Guideline CG74. Originally published October 2008, Updated February 2017. Available at: https://www.nice.org.uk/guidance/cg74/chapter/Key-priorities-for-implementation [accessed 6 March 2017].

Noah, N. (2006) *Controlling Communicable Diseases*. Maidenhead: Open University Press.

Nutland, W. and Cragg, L. (eds.) (2015) *Health Promotion Practice*, 2nd edn. London: Open University Press.

Semenza, J.C., Suk, J.E. and Tsolova, S. (2010) Social determinants of infectious diseases: a public health priority, *Eurosurveillance*, 15 (27): pii=19608.

Tanser, F., Barnighausen, T., Grapsa, E., Zaidi, J. and Newell, M.L. (2013) High coverage of ART associated with decline in risk of HIV acquisition in rural KwaZulu-Natal, South Africa, *Science*, 339 (6122): 966–971.

The Carter Center (2017) *Mali reports no guinea worm cases; disease remains in just three countries*, Press release, 11 January 2017. Available at: https://www.cartercenter.org/news/pr/guinea-worm-worldwide-cases-jan2017.html [accessed 5 March 2017].

UNAIDS (2010) *Combination HIV prevention: Tailoring and coordinating biomedical, behavioural and structural strategies to reduce new HIV infections*, Discussion paper. Geneva: UNAIDS. Available at:

http://www.unaids.org/en/resources/documents/2010/20101006_JC2007_Combination_
Prevention_paper.

Verelst, F., Willem, L. and Beutels, P. (2016) Behavioural change models for infectious disease
transmission: a systematic review (2010–2015), *Journal of the Royal Society Interface*, 13: 125.

Walker, T., Johnson, P.H., Moreira, L.A., Iturbe-Ormaetxe, I., Frentiu, F.D., McMeniman, C.J. *et al.* (2011)
The wMel *Wolbachia* strain blocks dengue and invades caged *Aedes aegypti* populations, *Nature*,
476 (7361): 450–453.

World Health Organization (WHO) (1986) *The Ottawa Charter for Health Promotion*. Available at: http://
www.who.int/healthpromotion/conferences/previous/ottawa/en/. [accessed 5 March 2017].

World Health Organization (WHO) (2004) *WHO Expert Consultation on Rabies, First report*, WHO technical
report Series 931. Geneva: WHO. Available at: http://www.who.int/rabies/trs931_%2006_05.pdf.

World Health Organization (WHO) (2009) *Natural ventilation for infection control in health-care settings*.
Geneva: WHO. Available at: http://www.who.int/water_sanitation_health/publications/natural_
ventilation.pdf.

World Health Organization (WHO) (2011) *Report on the burden of endemic health care-associated infection
worldwide*. Geneva: WHO. Available at: http://apps.who.int/iris/bitstream/10665/80135/1/
9789241501507_eng.pdf.

World Health Organization (WHO) (2014) *Post-exposure prophylaxis to prevent HIV infection*, Fact sheet.
Geneva: WHO. Available at: http://www.who.int/hiv/topics/prophylaxis/info/en/ [accessed
5 March 2017].

World Health Organization (WHO) (2015a) *Global technical strategy for malaria 2016–2030*. Geneva:
WHO. Available at: http://www.who.int/malaria/areas/global_technical_strategy/en/.

World Health Organization (WHO) (2015b) *Global Health Observatory (GHO) data: Under-five mortality*.
Available at: http://www.who.int/gho/child_health/mortality/mortality_under_five_text/en/
[accessed 5 March 2017].

World Health Organization (WHO) (2017) *International travel and health*. Geneva: WHO. Available at:
http://www.who.int/ith/mode_of_travel/communicable_diseases/en/.

Yakob, L. and Walker, T. (2017) Zika virus outbreak in the Americas: the need for novel mosquito control
methods, *The Lancet Global Health*, 4(3): e148–e149.

Zweigner, J., Magiorakos, A., Haag, L., Gebhardt, S., Meyer, E. and Gastmeier, P. (2013) *Systematic
review and evidence-based guidance on perioperative antibiotic prophylaxis*, ECDC technical
report. Stockholm: European Centre for Disease Prevention and Control. Available at: https://ecdc.
europa.eu/sites/portal/files/media/en/publications/Publications/Perioperative%20antibiotic%
20prophylaxis%20-%20June%202013.pdf.

7

Outbreak response

Liza Cragg

Overview

The previous three chapters have explored three essential components of communicable disease control: surveillance, prevention and vaccination. This chapter explains how these are applied in the event of an outbreak. The chapter starts by describing what outbreaks are and why they occur. It then explains why it is important to respond to outbreaks and who the key players in outbreak response are. The key stages of outbreak response are then described: preparing for an outbreak, investigating an outbreak, implementing measures to control the outbreak, and post-outbreak action. It concludes by explaining important factors in effective outbreak response.

Learning objectives

After reading this chapter, you will be able to:

- describe what outbreaks are and why they occur
- explain the key stages of outbreak response and the activities involved in each stage
- describe how to conduct an outbreak investigation
- explain the essential requirements for effective outbreak response

Key terms

Case definition: A set of criteria for deciding if an individual should be classified as having the health condition of interest.

Cluster: A group of cases in a defined place and/or time period that are suspected to be greater than the number of cases that would normally be expected, when the expected number may not be known.

Epidemic: The occurrence of more cases of disease than expected in a given area or among a specific group of people over a particular period of time.

> **Outbreak:**   Used as a synonym for epidemic. Can also be used to describe an epidemic limited to localized increase in the incidence of disease.
>
> **Pandemic:**   An epidemic that has spread to affect several countries over a large geographic region.

What are outbreaks and why do they occur?

An outbreak or epidemic is the occurrence of more cases of disease than would normally be expected in a given area, or among a specific group of people, over a particular period of time. The terms 'outbreak' and 'epidemic' are often used interchangeably, and there is generally no clear-cut distinction between the two, although the most common choice of term can sometimes depend on the context. For example, if the increase in cases is limited to localized area or source of infection, this will often be referred to as an outbreak, rather than an epidemic. Some organizations use outbreak, rather than epidemic, because it is considered to be less alarming for the public. In this book, epidemic and outbreak are used interchangeably. A number of cases in a defined place and/or time period that are suspected to be greater than the number that would normally be expected, when the expected number may not be known, is called a cluster. A cluster may be an early indication of an outbreak. Alternatively, an investigation may determine it is a due to sporadic and unrelated cases of the same disease or unrelated cases of similar but different diseases.

It is important to stress that there is no 'universal threshold' or minimum number of cases that can be applied across all contexts to define an outbreak or trigger an outbreak investigation. Even one single case of a communicable disease long absent from a population or caused by an infectious agent that has not previously been present in that community or area, or the emergence of a previously unknown disease, can constitute an event that warrants investigation.

A pandemic is an epidemic that has spread to affect several countries over a large geographic region. Pandemics typically involve the emergence of a virus (or strain of virus) that is new to humans, so very few people have immunity to it. For example, three influenza pandemics occurred in the twentieth century, one in 1918/19, one in 1957 and one in 1968 (Kilbourne, 2006). The most serious of these was the 1918/19 pandemic, which infected around one-third of the world's population and resulted in the deaths of between 50 and 100 million people globally.

How long an epidemic or pandemic continues depends on the disease characteristics and the action taken to respond to it. While some epidemics and pandemics of communicable disease last a relatively short time, others continue for many years. For example, the pandemic that began in the early

1980s continues today. More than 70 million people have been infected with the virus, of whom around 35 million have died (WHO, 2016a).

An epidemic of a communicable disease is usually the result of the inter-action of different factors. Chapter 2 looked at the role of the infectious agent, the susceptible host and the environment in causing communicable disease. A change in one or more of these can result in an epidemic. A new infectious agent may emerge in the human population, for example through zoonotic transmission or through mutation of an existing pathogen. Changes in the environment may also mean that infectious agents can spread to new geographical areas. For example, deforestation has been shown to increase the breeding areas of mosquitoes, leading to the introduction of mosquito-borne diseases to new areas (Kweka *et al.*, 2016). Changes in the behaviour of hosts can also contribute to outbreaks. For example, urbanization means cities are becoming important hubs for the transmis-sion of infectious diseases (Alirol *et al.*, 2011). Where new infectious agents emerge or existing ones spread to new areas, the exposed popula-tion will not have widespread immunity, so many people will be susceptible to infection, resulting in epidemics.

Epidemics can also result when control mechanisms break down for some reason. As Chapter 5 discussed, if vaccination coverage rates for a disease fall below the level required to ensure herd immunity, epidemics can rapidly re-emerge. Vaccination coverage rates may fall if people stop having confidence in a vaccine or if it stops being available. When a country experiences an emergency such as a natural disaster or armed conflict, services to prevent and control communicable disease, including surveil-lance, vaccination and treatment, can break down. At the same time, the affected population may be at increased risk of communicable disease because they are forced to move to areas with poor sanitation and housing.

There are some settings that are more prone to epidemics and where they may spread more quickly. These settings include places where people come together in close proximity and thus infectious agents are more likely to be transmitted, such as refugee camps, care homes, hospitals, prisons, schools and cruise ships. In some settings, people may also have an increased risk of exposure to infectious agents, for example hospitals. In addition, certain settings bring together people who are more likely to have increased susceptibility, including care homes for older people. In these settings, special attention needs to be given to preparing for outbreaks and responding to suspected outbreaks. More information about outbreaks in these settings is provided in the further reading section at the end of this chapter.

Epidemics are more likely to affect poor and vulnerable populations. The term 'infectious diseases of poverty' (IDoP) has been used to describe HIV, tuberculosis (TB), malaria and neglected tropical diseases (NTDs). This is because poor people are more likely to live in conditions that enable transmission, are less likely to have access to preventative and curative

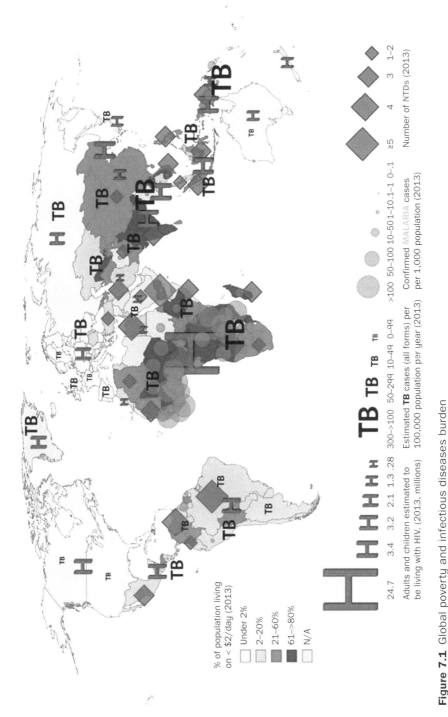

Figure 7.1 Global poverty and infectious diseases burden

Source: Reprinted from The Lancet, 63(1), Hansen, C. & Paintsil, E., Infectious Diseases of Poverty in Children: A Tale of Two Worlds, 37–66, Copyright (2016), with permission from Elsevier.

services, and are more likely to have other health conditions that make them more susceptible to infection. Infectious diseases of poverty primarily affect people in low-income countries. Figure 7.1 maps IDoP and the proportion of the population living on less than US$2 a day (Hansen and Paintsil, 2016). However, poor communities in high- and middle-income countries are also disproportionally affected by many epidemics. For example, research in Europe has found migrants and Roma communities are more at risk from epidemics of vaccine-preventable diseases (ECDC, 2013).

Low-income countries are most at risk of epidemics and bear the greatest burden of disease from epidemics (WHO, 2016b). They have limited resources for infrastructure that can prevent epidemics, including surveillance, preventative and curative health services, sanitation, housing and education services, legal and regulatory structures, and health systems. A greater proportion of their population lives in extreme poverty, which makes them more susceptible to infection and poor health outcomes. Low-income countries also have less capacity to identify and respond to outbreaks when they occur. In addition, outbreaks themselves further undermine fragile health systems and weak economies.

Why do outbreaks require a response?

There are several important reasons why urgent action needs to be taken to investigate and manage epidemics. First, it is important to take action to prevent the outbreak spreading, thus minimizing the number of people affected. If the source of the outbreak is contaminated food or water, it is important to find and remove the source to stop continued infection. If the source is an infected person or people, it is important to trace them and stop them transmitting the infection to others and take action to reduce the susceptibility of the population at risk if possible, for example through mass vaccination. Action to minimize the risk of outbreaks spreading across borders is also a requirement under the International Health Regulations, as will be discussed in more detail below.

Second, action is needed to limit the adverse impacts on the individuals and communities affected. This includes providing medical treatment to enable victims to recover, support to family members where victims have died, and resources to enable communities affected by a serious epidemic to rebuild economically and socially. Third, information gathered in responding to an epidemic is useful for preventing future outbreaks and improving prevention strategies. For example, investigating an epidemic of a vaccine-preventable disease may reveal that certain communities are not sufficiently immunized, so a catch-up vaccination campaign is needed. Fourth, outbreak investigations are an important way of generating new information about diseases. Indeed, investigating an outbreak can be the step in the discovery of a new infectious agent. Finally, outbreak response is an important way of addressing public concerns about a disease outbreak.

Key players in outbreak response

National governments are responsible for responding to outbreaks of communicable disease, as well as providing other health services to ensure the health and wellbeing of their populations. They do this through health systems, which must be adequately funded to meet the needs of the population. Chapter 10 of this book explores the role, characteristics and requirements of health systems in more detail. Most countries have a designated agency within the government health system that has specific responsibility for outbreak management. Governments in some countries work in collaboration with other international and national agencies to support their own capacities. Governments also play an essential role in preventing outbreaks by providing adequate social and environmental conditions, well-functioning health surveillance and accessible health care. Depending on the nature of the outbreak, other government agencies may need to be involved. For example, if the outbreak is linked to food, it is important the agency responsible for food safety and regulation is involved. Research institutes are also frequently involved in outbreak investigation and response.

Members of the public, patients, community groups and local representatives are also important players in outbreak response. They can provide key information that may be crucial to identifying the outbreak and its source. Outbreak response will require communicating with them to ensure that people can take any action necessary to minimize the risk of the outbreak spreading. In addition, outbreak response requires involving and communicating with a range of professionals. Who exactly is involved depends on the nature of the outbreak. Healthcare workers are likely to play an important role in identifying cases and treating infected people. Other professionals, such as teachers if children are affected, or people working in the food industry if it is a food-related outbreak, may also need to be involved.

It is important to engage with the full range of stakeholders early on or the outbreak response may lose the trust of the public. Without this trust, the public will not believe or act on the health information that is communicated by health authorities during an outbreak. It is also important to communicate proactively and at the outset, even if full information is not available, as the longer information is withheld, the more frightening it will seem when it is eventually revealed and a lack of information can generate rumours. Listening to and taking into account the perceptions, views and concerns of the public and other stakeholders is critical for the effectiveness of outbreak response. Chapter 8 looks at the role of communication in communicable disease control in more detail.

Governments have obligations to the broader international community as well as their own populations. The United Nations Committee on Economic, Social and Cultural Rights has recognized, 'given that some diseases are easily transmissible beyond the frontiers of a State, the international community has a collective responsibility to address this problem. The economically developed States Parties have a special responsibility and interest to assist the poorer developing States in this regard' (WHO, 2016c). The International Health Regulations (IHR) is an international legal instrument that is binding on all the countries in the world. Their aim is 'to prevent, protect against, control and provide a public health response to the international spread of disease in ways that are commensurate with and restricted to public health risks, and which avoid unnecessary interference with international traffic and trade' (WHO, 2016c). The WHO coordinates the IHR and helps countries to build capacities to detect, assess and report public health events through the Department of Global Capacities Alert and Response.

This department includes the Global Outbreak Alert and Response Network, a network of technical institutions that pool expertise and resources during response to outbreaks of international importance. The WHO also provides other support for outbreak response, including public health logistics, risk assessment, laboratory strengthening, travel health guidance to international organizations, training for medical and public health professionals, health systems' capacity for IHR, and guidance to countries on harmonizing their existing legal frameworks with IHR.

✎ Activity 7.1

Think about an outbreak that has recently affected your country. What caused the outbreak? What factors enabled it to spread? Who was responsible for managing the outbreak response? What did they do?

Feedback

There are lots of communicable diseases that regularly result in outbreaks and they have different causes. For example, you might have considered a measles outbreak that occurred when MMR vaccination rates dropped due to concerns about safety of the vaccine, or an outbreak of gastrointestinal illness as a result of food contamination. You might have considered an outbreak of influenza caused by a significant mutation in the virus, such as was seen with H1N1-pdm09 flu virus in 2009. Depending on where you live, you might have identified an outbreak of a vector-borne disease such as yellow fever, dengue fever or Zika. If you live in West Africa, you might have reflected on the outbreak of Ebola virus disease (EVD).

The list below provides some examples of national health authorities and agencies in different countries and international agencies with details of their websites where you can find information on how previous outbreaks were managed.

- England: Public Health England (PHE), https://www.gov.uk/topic/health-protection/infectious-diseases
- India: National Centre for Disease Control (NCDC), http://www.ncdc.gov.in
- South Africa: National Institute for Communicable Diseases, http://www.nicd.ac.za
- The United States: Centers for Disease Control and Prevention (CDC), https://www.cdc.gov/outbreaks/index.html
- Global: World Health Organization (WHO), http://www.who.int/csr/don/en/
- Europe: European Centre for Disease Prevention and Control (ECDC), http://ecdc.europa.eu/cdtr

Stages in outbreak management

There are several different stages in managing an outbreak, with each stage involving a number of activities, which are described below. It is important to stress that these stages, and the activities they are made up of, do not necessarily happen consecutively. Some activities need to be undertaken at the same time.

Preparing for an outbreak

Some activities need to happen before an outbreak begins. This is known as epidemic preparedness or outbreak preparedness. First, epidemic preparedness involves ensuring that the communicable disease surveillance system is in place and functioning properly. As explained in Chapter 4, one of the main objectives of this surveillance system is to act as an early warning system for potential outbreaks.

Second, epidemic preparedness involves producing an outbreak investigation and response plan. This should define which agencies are responsible for outbreak management, the criteria for undertaking an outbreak investigation, the composition of the outbreak response team, and the specific roles and responsibilities of organizations and positions in the team. Outbreak investigation requires a multidisciplinary team, including epidemiologists, laboratory specialists, clinicians and infection control personnel. Arrangements for consulting and information sharing at local and national levels also need to be explained. The plan should also identify different outbreak scenarios and how they will be managed. This means considering what type of outbreaks may occur in the setting or country concerned, how likely this is, what the impact could be and what needs to be done to prepare for it. The amount of resources dedicated to preparing for a particular scenario will depend on how likely it is and how serious its impact could be. An outbreak that could rapidly result in high mortality needs to be included in epidemic preparedness even if it is not considered very likely because the impact would be so significant. The outbreak investigation and response plan should ensure that the health system has sufficient capacity to respond to different epidemic scenarios and should identify this capacity. The information should be captured in an outbreak investigation and response plan, which needs to be prepared with the full participation of all stakeholders.

Third, epidemic preparedness requires information and training for those people who will be involved in outbreak investigation and response to ensure that they understand their role and how to fulfil it. In the event of an outbreak, there is very limited time so it is essential that staff are ready beforehand. This requires distributing and explaining the outbreak investigation and response plan and training staff on how to carry out the responsibilities it assigns to them. It also requires that protocols for investigating and treating diseases identified as outbreak scenarios are available and known to relevant staff.

Fourth, logistical preparations are required for epidemic preparedness. Reserve stocks of essential material should be available, such as vaccinations or medications. If it is not viable or cost-effective to purchase these in advance, it is important to identify a source from which they can be procured very quickly. Planning should also consider how resources should be mobilized and, if necessary, how patients should be prioritized or triaged, in order to optimize the use of available resources. In addition, it is important to identify in advance sites for isolation and treatment of infectious patients, laboratories that will be used to confirm cases, and transportation arrangements for patients and/or samples for diagnosis.

Investigating an outbreak

Potential outbreaks can be identified in different ways. Routine data collected through the surveillance system may indicate an increase in cases. A doctor who has seen a number of unusual cases in a short period of time may alert the local health department. A member of the public may report an incident they are concerned about, such as a family member becoming ill after eating food at an event or restaurant. When a health department is alerted about a potential outbreak, a decision is taken whether and how extensively to investigate based on criteria laid out in the outbreak investigation and response plan. These criteria will usually include factors such as the severity of the illness, the number of cases, the source, mode or ease of transmission, and the availability of prevention and control measures. Investigation is likely to be required if a suspected outbreak affects a large number of people, the disease is severe or the outbreak has the potential to affect others unless prompt control measures are taken.

For example, a single case of gastrointestinal illness is unlikely to require an investigation, but a cluster of cases may. The unusual presentation of a disease, a disease that is new or very rare, or a change in the pattern of disease in a particular area is likely to require investigation.

Outbreak investigations can involve different activities and methods depending on the organization leading the investigation, the resources available, the infectious agent, the number of cases, the perceived risk and public or political pressures.

There are, however, some steps that need to be taken in all outbreak investigations:

- *Prepare to investigate*: This will involve convening the outbreak investigation team, as outlined in the outbreak investigation and response plan. It may be necessary to review the scientific literature related to the disease in question. Depending on the disease and the population at risk, it may also be necessary to take some immediate control measures at this stage.
- *Establish the existence of an outbreak*: This involves checking that there are more cases than would normally be expected in the population and time period concerned. It requires reviewing incidence in the past in the area of the suspected outbreak over similar time periods, checking for recent changes in the surveillance system and in the population size, and exploring whether there are any contributory factors that might explain the apparent increase.
- *Confirm the diagnosis*: This requires a clinical description, obtaining medical and laboratory records of cases, and collection and testing of additional biological specimens if necessary and if possible.
- *Develop a case definition*: A case definition is a set of criteria that is used to determine whether an individual should be classified as having the health condition of interest (CDC, 2011). For an outbreak investigation, this typically includes clinical criteria and may also include restrictions on time, place and person. An important consideration when defining the case definition is to balance sensitivity with specificity. A more sensitive case definition (for example, anyone with at least one relevant symptom) will detect more cases, but is also likely to pick up individuals who are not true cases, such as people who have a different condition that causes some of the same symptoms. A more specific case definition, such as one based on laboratory confirmation, will identify true cases with much more certainty. However, such case definitions are likely to miss some true cases, for example due to limited laboratory capacity, or because specimens were not taken or were taken too late to detect the infectious agent. To help address these trade-offs between sensitivity and specificity, a case definition may include different categories of cases, such as confirmed (for example, based on laboratory analysis), probable (an individual who meets the clinical case definition, with supportive laboratory

results and/or epidemiological links to confirmed cases, but no definitive microbiological results) and suspected (some signs or symptoms but no laboratory confirmed diagnosis).

- *Case finding*: Case finding involves conducting a systematic search for cases based on the case definition. Depending on the circumstances, this can involve a range of approaches, such as examining available surveillance data, contacting health facilities to identify and collect information on additional cases, tracing and surveying those who may have been exposed to the suspected source(s) of the outbreak, and/or tracing the contacts of identified cases. It also requires developing what is known as a 'line listing' of cases. This is a spreadsheet with a separate line for each case, documenting information that should include: the name and/or ID number of the patient; clinical information such as the date of onset of symptoms, case status (confirmed, probable, suspected) and the outcome; demographic information such as age, ethnicity, gender; geographical area; and potential exposure information.

- *Perform descriptive epidemiology and generate hypotheses*: Descriptive epidemiology involves describing the outbreak over time through an epidemic curve, mapping the geographical location of cases, and calculating the population-based incidence by age and gender groups. It can also involve identifying the index cases, primary cases and secondary cases. These techniques are explained in more detail in Chapter 4 of this book and in *Introduction to Epidemiology,* which is part of the Understanding Public Health series (Carneiro and Howard, 2011). Figure 7.2 gives an example of a graph representing weekly and cumulative cases in a measles outbreak. It may also be necessary to conduct interviews with patients to try to find out what they have in common and undertake comparisons with similar outbreaks. This information can generate hypotheses about the outbreak. Hypotheses are predictive statements, which investigators develop from their analysis and interpretation of the data.

- *Evaluate and refine hypotheses*: Until proven otherwise, the hypothesis is merely an educated guess. The investigation team will need to evaluate the hypothesis by performing an epidemiological study. A cohort study looks at everyone who has been potentially exposed. A case-control study compares risk factors among those who meet the case definition with a selection of people who are not ill (controls).

- *Environmental studies*: Depending on the type of outbreak, it may also be necessary to undertake environmental studies to try to identify the source of the outbreak. This involves collecting food, water and/or environmental samples for analysis and determining whether and how contamination could have occurred.

- *Communicate findings*: The findings of all the above steps need to be written up in an outbreak investigation report that should be disseminated. The conclusions of the outbreak investigation report will be key for managing the outbreak.

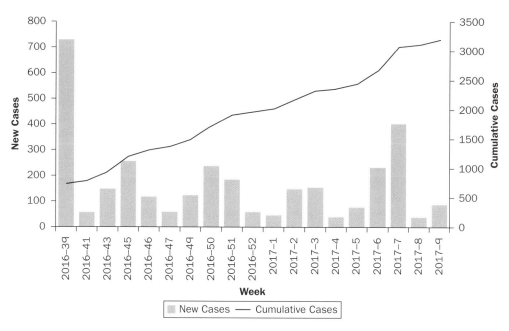

Figure 7.2 New measles cases by week of reporting

Source: ECDC (2017), http://ecdc.europa.eu/en/press/news/_layouts/forms/News_DispForm.
aspx?ID=1559&List=8db7286c-fe2d-476c-9133-18ff4cb1b568.

Implementing measures to control the outbreak

Controlling an outbreak includes a range of prevention and other activities intended to stop it spreading and reduce other negative impacts. It should be stressed that measures to control an outbreak should not be delayed until an outbreak investigation report is complete. Indeed, the investigation team needs to be involved in developing control measures throughout their research. Measures to control the outbreak will depend on the nature of the disease, the resources available, the population at risk and contextual factors. In general, they will focus on those parts of the chain of transmission that are amenable to intervention. They may include combinations of the vaccination and other prevention strategies outlined in Chapters 5 and 6 of this book. These are likely to be adapted to take account of the urgency of action in the case of an epidemic. They include:

- Communicating with the public – a lack of information leads to fear and rumours that can contribute to behaviours that will increase the spread of a disease or hinder control efforts. Depending on the disease and context, it may be necessary to formally declare an epidemic. Communication is discussed in more detail in Chapter 8 of this book.

- Enhancing the surveillance system for active case finding and more regular passive reporting. For example, during an outbreak, a surveillance system may require healthcare providers to submit details of suspected cases on a daily or weekly basis.
- Increasing access to diagnostic and treatment facilities so people who are infected can get treatment and limit their transmission to others.
- Temporary measures to limit mass gatherings or stop people coming together in ways that are likely to increase transmission, for example closing schools.
- Health promotion interventions to inform and empower people so they can minimize exposure to risk.
- Adopting or strengthening infection control precautions in the affected area and areas surrounding it.
- Measures to control the source and/or prevent exposure, such as removing a source of contaminated water and providing safe water to prevent cholera.
- Mass vaccination to increase the immunity of the at-risk population, for example to prevent measles.

Post-outbreak action

When an outbreak is over, there are a number of important actions that need to be taken:

- It is important to inform people that the outbreak is over and tell them if they need to continue with any actions to minimize the risk of further outbreaks.
- It is usually a good idea to carry out an evaluation of the outbreak management and to produce an end-of-epidemic report. This can help generate useful learning for future outbreak management and lessons to help avoid future outbreaks.
- Based on the experience of this outbreak, it may be useful to revisit the outbreak investigation and response plan, assess how well it worked in this outbreak and make any necessary changes.
- It is important to thank stakeholders, staff and the public for all their support in managing the outbreak. It is also important to extend solidarity and compassion to the affected populations.
- Additional services and support may be required for people affected. For example, where epidemics result in significant mortality, children whose parents have died may be left without primary caregivers.
- Disruption caused to usual health services as a result of the outbreak response efforts must be resolved and necessary action taken to restore preventative and curative services.

✎   **Activity 7.2**

Read the case study below and answer the questions that follow.

In the UK, following an organized open-water swimming event in the River Thames with 1100 competitors, the health agency responsible for managing outbreaks was made aware of cases of gastrointestinal illness among participants, including several severe cases.

1. Do you think this warrants an outbreak investigation?
2. If so, what would the objectives of the investigation be?
3. What methods would you use?

Feedback

1. This outbreak warrants an investigation because a large number of people participated in the event and several of the cases were serious. In addition, if the river was the source of the infection, other people using the river may be at risk of infection.

2. Potential objectives you may have considered include:

   • Describe the outbreak in terms of time, place and person, including plotting an epidemic curve of the number of cases by the date of symptom onset.
   • Obtain information on water quality of the river.
   • Obtain the results of any microbiological testing on samples submitted by outbreak cases.
   • Quantify the risk of illness among participants in the swimming race.
   • Identify factors associated with illness among swimmers.
   • Estimate the frequency of illness among respondents following previous open water swimming events.

3. Potential methods you may have considered include:

   • An environmental investigation of the microbiological quality of the water.
   • An epidemiological investigation, including: identifying and following up people who participated in the event as the study population to identify cases; a case definition of people who participated who experienced diarrhoea with symptom onset within 9 days of the event; the hypothesis that cases were more likely than non-cases to have ingested river water or greater quantities of river water.

More details are available in the report on which this case study is based (see PHE, 2012).

Factors in effective outbreak response

Outbreaks cannot always be prevented. However, previous experience and research has shown that prompt action can limit the spread of a disease and reduce its impact. Important factors that can influence the effectiveness of a response to an outbreak, whatever its nature, can be grouped into several themes. First, adequately funded health systems that are fair and accessible are essential. Capacities to detect potential outbreaks early and undertake an adequate response need to be an integral part of a well-functioning health system, including the integration of the private healthcare sector into the communicable disease surveillance system. Weak health systems can collapse when confronted with major epidemics, which mean people stop receiving or seeking health care for other diseases, like malaria, that cause more deaths yearly than the epidemic itself (WHO, 2015).

Second, outbreak preparedness makes a huge difference. For example, during the outbreak of EVD in 2014, countries like Nigeria, Senegal and Mali that had appropriate surveillance and laboratory support in place and took swift action were able to stop the virus before it gained a foothold (WHO, 2015).

Third, there is no one single intervention that can stop an epidemic by itself. Responding to an epidemic requires using different measures that work together to prevent new cases by breaking the chain of transmission. The type of measures depends on the biological, epidemiological and clinical characteristics of the disease, the population at risk, the resources available and other contextual factors.

Finally, community engagement is a critical factor for effective response to epidemics and outbreaks. Fear, rumours and misunderstanding spread quickly when accurate information is not available. This can contribute to behaviours that increase the risk of transmission. In addition, the cooperation and support of affected communities is an essential requirement for other control measures to be effective, such as vaccination, contact tracing, early reporting of symptoms, adherence to recommended protective measures and social distancing.

Activity 7.3

Read the case study below and answer the questions that follow it.

On 14th February 2003, the WHO reported 305 cases and two deaths of an unknown respiratory disease in Guangdong Province, China. On 21st February, a doctor from that province arrived in Hong Kong and stayed at the Metropole Hotel, unaware that he had been exposed to this unknown, respiratory pathogen and was now infected.

Between 18th and 21st February, a 78-year old woman was on vacation in Hong Kong with her husband – they stayed at the Metropole Hotel. Upon her return home to Toronto, Canada on 23rd February, she developed a fever, myalgia, sore throat and a cough. She was cared for by her family at her home. Over the next 10 days, her condition deteriorated and she died at home on 5th March.

On 27th February, this woman's 41-year old son (Case A) became ill with fever and respiratory symptoms. On 7th March, he presented to the emergency room (ER) of Hospital A and was admitted to the intensive care unit (ICU) where he died on 13th March. Between 3rd and 14th March, four more family members developed similar symptoms. The doctor who provided care to this family on 6th March developed respiratory symptoms 4 days later, on 10th March. By 19th March, several nurses who worked in the ER and ICU of Hospital A reported ill with fever and one or more of these symptoms: cough, malaise, myalgia and headache.

1. Is this an outbreak and does it warrant investigation?
2. What types of infectious agent could be the cause of an outbreak of respiratory illness?
3. In the early stages, are there any factors that might have made it difficult to identify if this was an outbreak?
4. What source(s) of routine surveillance data could help you confirm the existence of an outbreak in this investigation?

Feedback

1. This is an outbreak. It warrants investigation because the impacts are serious: a number of people have died and the cause of the disease is not known.
2. Respiratory illness can be caused by different types of infectious agents, including viruses, bacteria and fungi (although fungi are unlikely to present as an outbreak). These include viruses such as influenza A and B, rhinovirus, adenovirus and measles. Bacteria that cause respiratory symptoms include pertussis, tuberculosis and bacterial pneumonia, such as *Legionella*, *Streptococcus pneumoniae*, *Mycoplasma pneumonia* and *Chlamydia pneumoniae*.
3. Because respiratory infections often spread within a family, the situation was not initially defined as an outbreak. It was initially thought that the index case and her son (Case A) had TB. The family members were being investigated as potential TB case contacts. However, the two deaths and the rapid onset of respiratory symptoms among hospital staff raised suspicion that there was something going on unrelated to TB.

4. During respiratory disease outbreaks, laboratory surveillance data related to influenza and other reportable respiratory disease are useful. Epidemiologists can use these to verify baseline (expected) case counts, and may be able to identify unusual patterns/activity, leading or helping to confirm the existence of an outbreak. Systematic laboratory testing to identify the infectious agent is an important first step in any outbreak. In this scenario, while the causative agent was unknown, supplementary information from the laboratory helped rule out other diagnoses.

The information here has been taken from a case study developed by the WHO. As you may have realized, it is based on the early stages in the investigation of the outbreak of Severe Acute Respiratory Syndrome, caused by a new virus (the SARS coronavirus) that emerged in 2003 (WHO, 2007).

Summary

This chapter has explained what outbreaks are and why it is important to respond to suspected outbreaks rapidly. Effective outbreak response requires planning and preparation beforehand. The chapter also explained that investigating a suspected outbreak is essential for identifying how to control it effectively. It outlined the key steps involved in conducting an outbreak investigation and stressed it is important not to wait until an investigation is completed before putting in place control measures. The control measures used depend on the characteristics of the disease, the size of the population at risk, the resources available and other contextual factors. The chapter also emphasized the importance of effective health systems, communication and community engagement in outbreak response. The next section of this book discusses these aspects of communicable disease control in more detail.

Further reading

Centers for Disease Control and Prevention (CDC) (2016) *Outbreak investigations in healthcare settings*. Available at: https://www.cdc.gov/hai/outbreaks/ [accessed 14 March 2017].

Gregg, M.B. (1996) Conducting a field investigation, in M.B. Gregg (ed.) *Field Epidemiology* (pp. 44–59). Oxford: Oxford University Press.

Palmer, S.R. (1989) Epidemiology in search of infectious diseases: methods in outbreak investigation, *Journal of Epidemiology and Community Health*, 43: 311–314.

Public Health England (PHE) (2016) *Multi-agency contingency plan for the management of outbreaks of communicable diseases or other health protection incidents in prisons and other places of detention in England*. Available at: https://www.gov.uk/government/uploads/system/uploads/attachment_data/file/585671/multi_agency_prison_outbreak_plan.pdf [accessed 14 March 2017].

The Sphere Project (undated) *Humanitarian Charter and Minimum Standards in Humanitarian Response: Essential health services – control of communicable diseases standard 3: Outbreak detection and response*. Available at: http://www.spherehandbook.org/en/essential-health-services-control-of-communicable-diseases-standard-3-outbreak-detection-and-response/ [accessed 14 March 2017].

Ungchusak, K. (2002) Principles of outbreak investigation, in R. Detels, J. McEwen, R. Beaglehole and H. Tanaka (eds.) *Oxford Textbook of Public Health*, 4th edn. Oxford: Oxford University Press.

UNHCR (2011) *Epidemic preparedness and response in refugee camp settings: Guidance for public health officers*. Geneva: UNHCR. Available at: https://cms.emergency.unhcr.org/documents/11982/54561/UNHCR,+Epidemic+Preparedness+and+Response+in+Refugee+Camp+Settings,+2011+-/066ef592-d1bb-4059-a6dd-41900e4c8ade [accessed 14 March 2017].

References

Alirol, E., Getaz, L., Stoll, B., Chappuis, F. and Loutan, L. (2011) Urbanisation and infectious diseases in a globalised world, *Lancet Infectious Diseases*, 11 (2): 131–141.

Carneiro, I. and Howard, N. (2011) *Introduction to Epidemiology*. Maidenhead: Open University Press.

Centers for Disease Control and Prevention (CDC) (2011) *Principles of epidemiology in public health practice*, 3rd edn. Available at: https://www.cdc.gov/ophss/csels/dsepd/ss1978/ [accessed 14 March 2017].

European Centre for Disease Prevention and Control (ECDC) (2013) *Health inequalities, the financial crisis, and infectious disease in Europe*. Stockholm: ECDC.

European Centre for Disease Prevention and Control (ECDC) (2017) *Communicable disease threats report*, 5–11 March 2017, Week 10. Available at: https://ecdc.europa.eu/en/publications-data/communicable-disease-threats-report-5-11-march-2017-week-10 [accessed 20 March 2017].

Hansen, C. and Paintsil, E. (2016) Infectious diseases of poverty in children: a tale of two worlds, *Pediatric Clinics of North America*, 63 (1): 37–66.

Kilbourne, E.D. (2006) Influenza pandemics of the 20th century, *Emerging Infectious Diseases*, 12 (1): 9–14.

Kweka, E.J., Kimaro, E.E. and Munga, S. (2016) Effect of deforestation and land use changes on mosquito productivity and development in Western Kenya Highlands: implication for malaria risk, *Frontiers in Public Health*, 4: 238.

Public Health England (PHE) (2012) *Epidemiological investigation of an outbreak of gastrointestinal illness following a mass-participation swim in the River Thames, London, October 2012*. Available at: https://www.gov.uk/government/uploads/system/uploads/attachment_data/file/331702/ThamesSwim-epidemiological_report_on_outbreak_of_gastrointestinal_illness.pdf [accessed 14 March 2017].

World Health Organization (WHO) (2007) *Case study: An outbreak with respiratory symptoms, Toronto, Canada*. Available at: http://www.who.int/ihr/lyon/surveillance/case_studies/en/ [accessed 14 March 2017].

World Health Organization (WHO) (2015) *Strategic response plan: West Africa Ebola outbreak*. Available at: http://apps.who.int/iris/bitstream/10665/163360/1/9789241508698_eng.pdf?ua=1&ua=1 [accessed 12 January 2018].

World Health Organization (WHO) (2016a) *Global Health Observatory (GHO) data for HIV/AIDS for 2015*. Geneva: WHO. Available at: http://www.who.int/gho/hiv/en/ [accessed 14 March 2017].

World Health Organization (WHO) (2016b) *Guidance for managing ethical issues in infectious disease outbreaks*. Geneva: WHO. Available at: http://apps.who.int/iris/bitstream/10665/250580/1/9789241549837-eng.pdf [accessed 14 March 2017].

World Health Organization (WHO) (2016c) *International Health Regulations (2005)*, 3rd edn. Geneva: WHO. Available at http://www.who.int/ihr/publications/9789241580496/en/ [accessed 9 February 2017].

SECTION 3

Application of measures to control communicable disease

.

Communication and communicable disease control

Will Nutland

Overview

Communication is at the heart of any communicable disease control strategy. How and when health professionals communicate with the public, the language they use, and the communication methods they employ, will impact on how the public engage and respond. This chapter outlines the importance of good communication in the application of communicable disease control, and describes proactive and reactive responses. It highlights the role of mass and social media and introduces some of the most commonly used methods of communication such as press releases, press conferences, media interviews, case studies, and communication outreach to key communities. The chapter explains some of the key features of effective communication, including some of the commonly used techniques for communicating uncertainty and risk.

Learning objectives

After reading this chapter, you will be able to:

- understand the importance of communication as part of communicable disease control
- explain the difference between reactive and proactive communication responses
- explain the principles of a communication strategy as part of outbreak response
- describe some of the key methods and approaches in communicating as part of communicable disease control
- understand some of the key features that support effective communication

Key terms

Communications strategy: A plan outlining the actions that will be taken, including the communication methods, the intended target groups, and the key information and actions that are intended to be released.

Off-the-record: Information provided, usually to a journalist, that the informant does not wish to be publicly reported or attributed to them.

On-the-record: Information provided, usually to a journalist, that the informant states can be publicly reported and attributed to them, including official or public statements.

Proactive response: A response that is made when attempting to 'push' a news story.

Reactive response: A response that is made once a news story is already in the public domain.

Communication and communicable disease

Communication is an essential element of communicable disease control strategies. Health professionals have a role and a duty to provide facts and information to the public about communicable diseases, as well as ways of preventing or containing them. This can often involve providing reassurance or a warning about the relative risk of a communicable disease (for example, that a particular disease is hard to transmit, or is confined to a very small proportion of a population). It also frequently involves outlining what actions authorities are taking to control a disease (for example, a vaccination programme, or a health promotion intervention). This is even more important during periods of disease outbreaks and, as shown in Chapter 7, developing a communications strategy will be central to any outbreak control group. Communication expertise is now considered to be as essential to outbreak and disease control as other skills, such as epidemiological expertise and laboratory analysis (WHO, 2005). There are different situations in which proactive and reactive communication or a combination of the two is required, including informing the public about control and prevention strategies, responding to public concerns and managing outbreaks. These are discussed in more detail below.

Proactive and reactive communications

How issues around communicable disease are communicated will depend on whether a proactive or reactive response is taken. Proactive responses are broadly driven when health professionals are actively seeking to 'push' a health story into the public domain. For example, a new vaccine programme might be about to launch in a particular setting, or new data on the outcomes of a recent communicable disease control intervention might have become available. In such circumstances, commonly used approaches might be: to issue a report, a press release or a statement; to organize a press conference, often with panels of experts to respond to questions; or to arrange an interview with a relevant and influential media outlet. Reactive approaches are more likely to be employed when health professionals have to respond to health stories over which they have little control. For example, rumours of an outbreak might have been reported in the press before it was confirmed, or data might have been published without accurate analysis. In recent years, with the predominance of 24-hour news coverage and social media, information on outbreaks and other health issues can spread at an unprecedented pace – and may not always be accurate. As such, it is increasingly important to have a timely and effective reactive response to both mainstream and social media coverage.

Communication during outbreaks

Health issues more commonly become a news story if the issue is seen to be unusual or unexplained, if there is a perception of fear or risk to life, if it has a disproportionate impact on a particular demographic group, or if it has a political or economic dimension. Fast-moving stories, such as the rapid development of a communicable disease across a population, are also more likely to be picked up by news media.

When outbreaks of communicable disease occur, therefore, they often hit the headlines, especially if they impact disproportionately on a sub-population or if there is uncertainty about how the disease is transmitted. As public health professionals, it is important to recognize that the media might have a vested interest in sensationalizing a disease or an outbreak. Gardner (2008) notes how during an outbreak of variant Creutzfeldt–Jakob disease (vCJD), a rare and fatal human neurodegenerative condition linked to eating beef that first occurred in the UK in 1996, journalists coined the phrase 'mad cow disease'. That term was seen to give the infection a less abstract and more emotive label, possibly leading to more people avoiding beef consumption than when more scientific terminology was used. However, it also gave rise to reporting that had the potential to misinform the public. Indeed, vCJD illustrates how the novelty of new and poorly understood diseases can be captured by the media in ways that are both beneficial and challenging. Such new and poorly understood diseases receive enormous coverage and attention, albeit for relatively short periods of time, while ongoing diseases, that have a much greater toll on the population, can be neglected or ignored. Researchers at the King's Fund (Gardner, 2008) developed a 'death-per-news-story' ratio and found just 0.33 deaths from vCJD for every BBC news story about the disease. However, there were over 8500 smoking-related deaths for every BBC news story about smoking.

Communication guidelines for outbreaks

The WHO (2005) has identified five key best practice principles for communication during an outbreak. When implemented, the principles are intended to increase public resilience and guide public action to support containment of an outbreak. These guidelines are:

- *Trust*: The overarching goal of outbreak communication is to communicate in ways that build, maintain and restore trust. Evidence demonstrates that the less the public trusts those who are supposed to protect them, the more alarmed the public will be and the less likely they will be to engage with outbreak management interventions.
- *Announcing early*: Parameters of trust are established in the outbreak's first announcement. As such, its timing, candour and detail are important. Information about outbreaks cannot be kept hidden and doing so can lead to rumours and misinformation. Delaying disclosure of information can lead to overestimation of risk, and can make information seem more frightening when it is eventually disclosed. Early announcements of information are often based on incomplete information. Where announcements include incomplete information, this should be acknowledged and it should be stated that information is likely to change over time.
- *Transparency*: Maintaining trust requires transparency, including making data, risk-assessment plans and decision-making processes public. Transparency demonstrates that public health professionals are seeking answers and have processes in place. Within this there is a balance to strike between the rights of individuals. While being transparent, it is important to respect patient confidentiality, so communication should be about cases and not about individual patients.
- *The public*: Understanding the public is essential to communicating effectively. Crisis communication should be about dialogue, rather than telling the public what they should do or think. Public concerns should be appreciated and validated. Public views that are incorrect should be acknowledged and corrected – not ignored or dismissed. Risk communication should include information about what people can do themselves to protect their own health and safety.
- *Planning*: Decisions and actions of public health officials can have more effect on trust and public risk perception than communication. In other words, the public pays more attention to what public health officials do than what they say. Therefore, it is essential to have a risk communication plan in place in advance of outbreaks. This should include communication planning that acknowledges uncertainty and empathizes with the public's beliefs and fears. It should also have a clear plan for which agencies and individuals are responsible for each communication role and how they will carry this out.

Case study 8.1

In 2015, a dentist in Wales, UK was suspended from dental practice after it was discovered that there was poor infection control practice in his dental surgery. After a colleague raised concerns about the dentist's poor infection control practice, the health authority made a decision to contact all patients of the dental surgery. Over 3000 letters were sent out but the health authority admitted that thousands of other people, who had been previous patients at the dental surgery, could not be contacted. Although there was no evidence of blood-borne infection as a result of the actions of the dentist, the authority stated that they had a duty to protect and inform the public, and that they should be transparent about their concerns. A temporary telephone advice line was established, and concerned individuals were offered blood tests if they wanted them. Current and former patients of the dental surgery were given reassurance that there was a very low risk of having become infected with a blood-borne disease as a result of treatment at this dental surgery.

 Activity 8.1

In the case study above, the health authority stated that it wanted to be transparent about its concerns. What might be the communication benefits and challenges of being transparent around a potential communicable disease control issue?

Feedback

In this instance, the health authority followed WHO best practice and candidly informed the public about the situation. The WHO (2005) states that public panic is rare when the public is informed about an outbreak. By being open and transparent, the health authority was able to reach thousands of people who might have been exposed to a blood-borne infection. Had the authority decided to be less candid, there might have been accusations of a 'cover up' and this might have undermined public trust. Indeed, by being proactive, the authority avoided the need for a potential future reactive response. For example, if the colleague had felt their concerns were not being taken seriously by the health authority, they might have contacted the press directly. The challenge of a widespread media strategy is that people who have not been exposed, or have been to another dental surgery in the neighbouring area, might be alarmed or concerned. This was mitigated by naming the dental surgery and by providing advice that the risk of infection via the surgery was very low. Further, a phone helpline provided further information and advice.

The role of mass media and social media

Mass media is a common way of communicating with the public about health in general and about disease control specifically. Mass media has historically played a significant role in determining how communicable diseases are perceived by the public and how the public engages with disease prevention. It includes television, radio, billboards and print media in newspapers and magazines. Communicable disease control strategies, including vaccination programmes, prevention and outbreak control, are addressed in Chapters 5, 6 and 7. Mass media can play a role in all of these. However, there are strengths and limitations to using mass media. The chapter 'Using mass media to promote health' in the book *Health Promotion Practice* (Nutland and Cragg, 2015), part of the Understanding Public Health series, provides a more in-depth exploration of these strengths and limitations.

In addition to the educational role mass media can play in explaining what causes disease and how people can protect themselves, it also has a norm functioning and socialization effect. Finnegan and Viswanath (1997) identify this 'norm sending' role and argue that ongoing interaction with the media can influence how an audience views or responds to a health issue. As such, a health promoter has the potential to shape how people think about a health issue and their related behaviour by influencing what is seen and shown in the media. This might involve the health promoter engaging with a journalist to influence how health issues are addressed through news stories, or contributing to contents of radio and television broadcasts, including fictional programmes.

Social media are 'web-based technologies and services that allow end users to interact and collaborate as content creators, rather than the one-way information flow on relatively static . . . websites' (Gold *et al.*, 2012). Social media is increasingly being used to communicate around health, and communicable disease control in particular. Social media sites such as Facebook, Twitter and YouTube have facilitated relatively cheap and peer-driven ways of communicating, and increasing numbers of health organizations and institutions now use social media to communicate to their target audiences. User data enables geographically targeted or population-based advertising, enabling health communications to be highly targeted and tailored. In addition, the proliferation of mobile phone apps has led to targeted geographical location services that enable individuals within a specific area to be targeted with a specific communication. This has multiple possible uses for communicable disease control, including: to invite a specific population group to attend a clinical service for a vaccination; to deliver a specific communication to those of a particular age or gender, such as a reminder about hand washing; or to provide individuals attending a specific venue, area or region with specific information in an outbreak scenario.

The use of social media to communicate health information is not without its challenges, not least the dearth of evidence of the impact of social media on health outcomes (Nutland, 2015). Additionally, concerns around confidentiality and privacy might dissuade sub-populations that could most benefit from a health intervention from encountering them on social media (Witzel et al., 2016), especially if the health issue is stigmatized. Given the participatory dimension of social media content being created and driven by users themselves, a further challenge of social media is navigating information that is inaccurate, especially given recent concerns regarding 'fake news'.

Methods used in communicating about communicable disease control

As detailed above, the methods used to communicate around communicable disease will be driven by whether a proactive or reactive response is needed. There is a broad range of methods that can be used in communicable disease communication, and these are described below.

Press releases

A press release is a concise statement, often as short as one page, about a particular issue that frequently includes a quote from one or more influential people. Press releases have the advantage of being able to provide 'top-level' information on a communicable disease to a broad media audience, and journalists can build a story around the details given in the release. Press releases might be intended to 'stand-alone', with no further information being given or being available, but more usually they will be a 'hook' for journalists to use to glean further information and details. If a press release is being used proactively to launch a report, for example, it will include a link to the report or the summary of the report. If a press release is being used in response to a crisis or emergency situation, it might include details of helplines, or key information on actions that the public can take to avoid infection or to access treatment. Press releases should be concise, jargon-free and engaging; news journalists will receive dozens every day, so a press release needs to capture their attention. A press release should include the contact details of a person who can provide further details, such as the press office of the organization issuing the release.

Press conferences

A popular method of communicating health issues to the media is to hold a press conference. These are meetings to announce significant news to a body of journalists so they can publish articles on the health issue. Press conferences have the advantage of ensuring that all media are seen to be getting access to the same information and that information is provided in a controlled environment. Press conferences also reduce the need to do one-on-one interviews. However, because they are 'on-the-record' meetings, they can also be highly pressured, with the possibility that difficult or complex questions will be asked by attending journalists, and with the potential for those providing the information being misquoted or challenged in ways that are unplanned or unexpected. Health professionals that are experienced with dealing with the press will have developed strategies to mitigate against such risks, including preparing a set of key questions, and responses to them; sticking to facts and refusing to provide conjecture; and delivering a pre-prepared short statement to the press.

Media interviews

A further way of communicating about communicable disease control is through media interviews. Interviews can be a powerful way of providing reassurance and information to key populations. In some circumstances, a trusted and reliable journalist might be used to 'break' a news story by reporting it for the first time, with a guarantee of an exclusive interview before the information is shared more broadly. This has an advantage of the news being released with an element of control and accuracy. It also has the potential to backfire if other journalists consider that they have had the information withheld from them. Public health professionals are commonly trained in undertaking media interviews and to know and understand the pitfalls and challenges of live or recorded interviews. The UK's Science Media Centre provides useful and beneficial tips for communicating science to the media (Science Media Centre, 2013).

Case studies

Providing case studies as part of press releases, press conferences and interviews can be a powerful way of providing tangible, real-world experiences that the target audience can identify with. Personal stories are commonly used to draw an emotional response from the audience but care is needed to ensure that the specifics of a case study do not detract from the key information being communicated or undermine that communication. For example, having a case study of someone taking part in a vaccination programme in a clinic in a city centre, might only resonate with those who can access urban clinics. This might have an unintended consequence that those living in suburban or rural areas see the vaccination for urban dwellers only.

Outreach by peers and community organizations

Not all populations will have access to, or be able to benefit from, the communication methods above. Potential barriers include: lack of access to printed news media, television or other media technologies; unfamiliarity with the language that the information is being provided in; visual or hearing impairment, and illiteracy. Direct contact interventions may need to be used in conjunction with the methods above. This includes undertaking communication activities with or directly through non-government organizations (NGOs), community leaders and community groups. It may require building peer capacity to undertake outreach that informs and educates people about communicable disease. Using mixed methods of communication will strengthen its reach and health authorities should not assume that a passive approach (for example, relying on a press release) will be sufficient to communicate with and reach key populations.

Factors for effective communication on communicable disease

The sections above have focused on the purpose and methods of communication on communicable disease issues. *How* these communication methods are used is crucial to their effectiveness. This section discusses some critical factors for effective communication, including: communicating with a lay audience; using data, percentages and numbers; and communicating uncertainty and risk.

Communicating with a lay audience

Medical professionals and public health experts are used to using technical terminology when referring to and discussing their work. Pinker (1994) refers to 'the curse of knowledge': the concept that an expert may be unable to imagine that other people do not know what that expert knows. In any communications targeted at the public and those who are not experts in the field of communicable disease, it is essential to use language and terminology that is understandable and unambiguous. Freeman (2014) identifies a range of words and phrases commonly used by medical professionals and scientists that will have a different meaning to patients or lay audiences. These include 'determine', 'significant', 'fraction', 'trauma', 'fate' and 'predict'. As such, it is important when developing any communications strategy to consider carefully the words, phrases and terminology used. Avoiding jargon, acronyms or measurements that the public will not understand is important. One good rule of thumb is to ask several members of the target audience, who are not experts in the field, to read through any communication before it is released, to check for ambiguity or words or phrases that may be unclear, misleading or confusing.

Data, numbers and percentages

It is natural for public health professionals and other scientists to communicate information using data, numbers and percentages because most scientific research relies on quantitative analysis. However, Blastland and Dilnot (2008) highlight how the tendency to use percentages to illustrate the potential health impact of undertaking a particular action leads to widespread confusion. To illustrate their point, they use an example of a large report from the World Cancer Research Fund that stated that eating an extra ounce of bacon a day increased the risk of colorectal cancer by 21%. It is easy to see how such a statement might be misunderstood, especially at any individual level because most people interpret this to mean, 'if I eat extra bacon every day, I'll increase my chance of getting cancer by 21%'. Blastland and Dilnot (2008) show how media coverage of this report conflated and confused the research even further, with little acknowledgement of the understanding of baseline risk of colorectal cancer. Usefully, they suggest that a better way of communicating the risk from this research is as follows:

> About five men in a hundred typically get colorectal cancer in a lifetime. If they all ate an extra couple of slices of bacon every day, about six would.
>
> (p. 110)

Blastland and Dilnot conclude that counting people, rather than stating relative percentages, instantly makes the data more understandable and puts it into perspective.

Communicating uncertainty and risk in communicable disease

One of the biggest challenges in communicating about communicable disease is that, especially in an outbreak context, it is likely public health experts will not have complete information and the situation will develop and change rapidly. For example, the cause of an illness may be unknown, at least initially, and the numbers of people affected by an outbreak can increase very quickly. Not having complete, accurate and up-to-date details on a communicable disease outbreak might be unsettling for the public. However, providing false or vague information can undermine public trust in an outbreak response. The UK's Science Media Centre (SMC) provides a template of short, easy-to-remember statements, known as soundbites, that scientists and public health professionals can use when communicating uncertainty, including responses to questions such as: Why don't you have an answer?, Why do scientists disagree?, and Why does evidence in one small study appear to contradict that of other studies? (Science Media Centre, 2012).

In addition, a medical or public health professional may perceive a potential public health risk and action to address that risk very differently from the public, or a sub-population of the public. This chapter has already addressed how risk or danger can be communicated more clearly by using data or examples that are tangible and understandable. It is also important to understand that some communities – including those living with ongoing risks and challenges in their lives – might not share the same view or perception of risk as the population as a whole. However risks are perceived, there is a growing consensus that the public has a right to information that is clear and not misleading, with calls for medical professionals, scientists and others to subscribe to ethical policies that report risks clearly and unambiguously (Gigerenzer, 2002; Hofman and Au, 2017).

Activity 8.2

For each of the scenarios described below, outline the type of communication strategy you might employ:

1. A seasonal flu vaccination programme in a high-income country
2. A periodic campaign to encourage correct use of long-lasting insecticide-treated nets to prevent malaria
3. An outbreak of hepatitis A in men who have sex with men (MSM) in New York City
4. An outbreak of measles in a small town
5. An outbreak of meningitis in a student college community

Feedback

Your communication strategy should be guided by whether a proactive or reactive response is necessary. In the first two scenarios, the response will be proactive, allowing for research and evidence to guide the communication strategy, including evaluation of past communication strategies. Press releases, press conferences and broad population media communications are likely to be used, possibly with additional geographical or sub-population targeting.

In the third scenario of a hepatitis A outbreak among MSM in New York City, it is likely that you would use a more sensitive and nuanced communications strategy. Highly targeted media or social media interventions might be more effective than issuing broad public statements, especially if the outbreak is relatively contained.

For the fourth scenario of a measles outbreak in a small town, the communications strategy again needs be highly targeted. Children who are unvaccinated will be most at risk, so it will be important to communicate with parents and guardians to provide specific information outlining the importance of vaccination and the evidence of its safety. You might consider such an outbreak as an opportunity to communicate more widely in the area or region about childhood vaccination and reinvigorate vaccination programmes locally.

In the fifth scenario of an outbreak of meningitis in a student college community, the initial communication strategy might depend on how contained the outbreak is. Communicating directly with the student body using social media and posters might be more efficient and effective than, for example, issuing a press release. The communication strategy might need to include a larger and wider audience if there are concerns about the impact of the outbreak on the surrounding population. Again, this might serve as an opportunity to communicate more generally about the availability and importance of pre-college vaccination programmes.

In all of the above, careful thought has to be given to the impact of any communications strategy on vulnerable and marginalized communities.

Summary

Communicating about communicable disease cannot be an afterthought: it needs to be central to any communicable disease control and outbreak response strategy. This means communication is a key skill for public health and communicable disease experts. There is a broad range of methods and approaches that can be used to communicate about communicable disease. However, care and attention is needed to ensure that the methods used will reach the target audiences, including the public as a whole, as well as key sub-populations. Communication must be clearly understandable and use appropriate language. Uncertainty and risk must be communicated thoughtfully and sensitively. Planning for communication as part of an outbreak response needs to be undertaken in advance. The WHO communication principles provide a useful framework for positioning and developing communication strategies for communicable disease control and outbreak response.

References

Blastland, S. and Dilnot, A. (2008) *The Tiger that Isn't: Seeing Through a World of Numbers*. London: Profile Books.

Finnegan, J.R. and Viswanath, K. (1997) Communication theory and behaviour change, in K. Glanz, F.M. Lewis and B.K. Rimer (eds.) *Health Behavior and Health Education*, 2nd edn. San Francisco, CA: Jossey-Bass.

Freeman, T. (2014) *Physician, explain thyself: Science English vs lay English*. Available at: https://stroppy editor.wordpress.com/2014/11/27/physician-explain-thyself-science-english-vs-lay-english/ [accessed 3 July 2017].

Gardner, D. (2008) *Risk: The Science and Politics of Fear*. London: Virgin Books.

Gigerenzer, G. (2002) *Reckoning with Risk*. London: Penguin.

Gold, J., Pedrana, A.E., Stoone, M.A., Chang, S., Howard, S., Asselin, J. *et al.* (2012) Developing health promotion interventions on social networking sites: recommendations for the FaceSpace Project, *Journal of Medical Internet Research*, 14 (1): e30.

Hofman, M. and Au, S. (2017) *The Politics of Fear – Médecins Sans Frontières and the West African Ebola Epidemic*. Oxford: Oxford University Press.

Nutland, W. (2015) Using media to promote health: mass media, social media, and social marketing, in W. Nutland and L. Cragg (eds.) *Health Promotion Practice*, 2nd edn. Maidenhead: Open University Press.

Nutland, W. and Cragg, L. (eds.) (2015) *Health Promotion Practice*, 2nd edn. Maidenhead: Open University Press.

Pinker, S. (1994) *The Language Instinct*. London: Penguin.

Science Media Centre (2012) *Top tips for media work*. London: Science Media Centre. Available at: http://www.sciencemediacentre.org/wp-content/uploads/2012/09/Top-Tips-2012.pdf

Science Media Centre (2013) *Communicating uncertainty in a sound bite*. London: Science Media Centre. Available at: https://inspiringsa.org.au/wp-content/uploads/2016/06/publications-ASMC-Uncertainty-2012.pdf

Witzel, T.C., Guise, A., Nutland, W. and Bourne, A. (2016) It Starts With Me: privacy concerns and stigma in the evaluation of a Facebook health promotion intervention, *Sexual Health*, 13 (3): 228–233.

World Health Organization (WHO) (2005) *WHO outbreak communication guidelines*. Geneva: WHO. Available at: http://www.who.int/csr/resources/publications/WHO_CDS_2005_28/en/

Ethics and communicable disease control

Will Nutland

Overview

Anyone involved in the application of communicable disease control will need to make decisions about how to act. Those decisions should be informed by ethical principles that provide a framework through which to make an ethical analysis. Practitioners will inevitably have to weigh up the benefits and costs of privileging one ethical principle over another. This chapter explores fundamental principles of ethics, including those specifically for public health practice and the application of communicable disease control. The chapter concludes with an analysis of how responses to communicable disease control can be driven by fear, and the ethical consequences of fear-driven approaches.

Learning objectives

After reading this chapter, you will be able to:

- explain a range of key and commonly used principles of ethics and how they might be applied to public health and communicable disease control
- understand the challenges and tensions of prioritizing different ethical principles in practice
- understand how fear can drive communicable disease control decisions that are counterproductive and the implications of fear-driven approaches to working with communities
- understand a specific example of contemporary ethical challenges in communicable disease control

Key terms

Beneficence: The concept that we have an obligation to bring about good in all our actions and must take positive steps to prevent harm.

Ethics: Moral principles that guide a person's behaviour or how an activity is conducted.

> **Non-maleficence:** The principle that we should do no harm to others and we should strive to minimize any harm when harm cannot be avoided.
>
> **The Siracusa Principles:** International principles established in 1985 that determine the limitations and appropriateness of limiting key fundamental human rights.

Ethics

Why is it important to consider ethics in communicable disease control?

There are numerous approaches that can be used to influence decisions about communicable disease control and public health in general. The approaches used will depend on the political and value frameworks under which the individual, organization, government or other authority concerned acts or operates. It is possible to achieve public health or communicable disease control objectives by coercive means, including: forced removal or migration of populations; quarantine, imprisonment or refusal of entry to individuals or key groups at borders; mandatory testing and vaccination or treatment without individual consent; exclusion zones and travel bans; and restrictions on social or sexual mixing between groups of people. Although such approaches might 'work' to varying degrees, it is questionable if the restrictions on individual freedoms and rights can be justified by the public health outcomes. Questioning the ethics of approaches used in public health should be fundamental to any application of communicable disease control. In addition, not only are some practices ethically questionable, the damage that they might cause to public confidence in health authorities might mean that the public will not trust those authorities in the future.

Ethical principles

Applying ethical principles

Ethical principles provide a framework and a lens through which to apply public health practice. Applying these principles involves a process of ethical analysis. That is, identifying relevant principles, applying them to relevant situations, and then weighing up those principles against each other in circumstances when those principles might be seen to be in competition (WHO, 2016).

Fundamental principles of ethics

Beauchamp and Childress (1989) describe four fundamental principles that assist in determining whether a decision in biomedicine is ethical or not. These are:

- *The principle of respect for autonomy* – that we should respect the decisions made by others about how they lead their lives and the choices they make.
- *The principle of beneficence* – that we have an obligation to bring about good in all our actions and must take positive steps to prevent harm.
- *The principle of non-maleficence* – that we should do no harm to others and we should strive to minimize any harm when harm cannot be avoided.
- *The principle of justice* – that we should treat everyone equally, with fairness and impartially.

Ethical principles for public health

Schröder-Bäck *et al.* (2014) propose seven principles of ethics for public health, building on the four fundamental principles above. They make the case that, while each principle should be conceived of as being prima facie (that is, of equal weight) at the outset of moral deliberation, through deliberation one or more principles may emerge as having greater or lesser importance than others. The seven principles they identify are:

- *Non-maleficence* – the principle that one should do no harm. This principle is related to the commonly understood Hippocratic principle of medical ethics – first of all, do no harm. Schröder-Bäck *et al.* (2014) argue that in policy and practice, there are likely to be times when degrees of harm are 'traded off' between occasions when greater harm can be avoided or when there is a greater benefit that can be obtained.
- *Beneficence* – the principle that one should bring about good or bring about benefits in one's actions. This principle is related to the Hippocratic principle that physicians should heal and help their patients.
- *Health maximization* – Schröder-Bäck *et al.* (2014) argue that even when following non-maleficence and beneficence, it does not necessarily follow that health maximization is brought about. This principle raises one of the possible tensions between more traditional biomedical principles of ethics and principles of ethics that may be applied to public health – and, therefore, by default – to communicable disease control. Public health is concerned with improving the health of a population, whereas biomedicine is concerned with the health of individuals. Consequently, the improvement of population health might conflict with the two principles articulated above for the health of individuals.

- *Efficiency* – this principle establishes that public health professionals have a moral duty to ensure that health resources are used efficiently. This is even more important given that all health systems will have more health need than resources available.
- *Respect for autonomy* – this principle acknowledges that every person has a value of their own. Given public health's focus on population-wide benefits, there is potential for the rights of and respect for individuals to be lost. This principle raises an obvious tension: when and in what circumstances might it be appropriate to override the autonomy of an individual, for the benefit of a greater public health good?
- *Justice* – this principle sets out that there should be equality of opportunity and a fair distribution of health outcomes across society. This is often described in public health as 'health equity'.
- *Proportionality* – Schröder-Bäck *et al.* (2014) acknowledge that this final principle differs from the six preceding ones because it is a normative principle; that is, it is a principle that states how things ought to be done. This principle states that any restriction of individual freedoms for broader public health good must be proportional and that positive outcomes must be weighed up against any negative ones.

Ethical principles for communicable disease outbreaks

The World Health Organization (WHO, 2016) has developed guidance on managing ethical considerations around communicable disease outbreak responses that build upon ethical principles of public health. These seven principles are laid out in Table 9.1.

As the frameworks described above demonstrate, there is no universal set of ethical principles that are applied to public health and communicable disease control. Institutions and organizations will have principles upon which their staff will be expected to act, and scenarios and circumstances in which one or more principle might be seen as more important than another. However, the WHO has prepared guidance to support governments on communicable disease control. This guidance refers to the Siracusa Principles that were adopted by the United Nations Economic and Social Council in 1984 (United Nations Economic and Social Council, 1984). The WHO guidance (2016: 9) states that:

> . . . in balancing competing principles during infectious disease outbreaks, countries must respect their obligations under human rights agreements . . . The Siracusa Principles provide that any restrictions on human rights must be carried out in accordance with the law and in pursuit of a legitimate objective of general interest . . . such restrictions must be strictly necessary and there must be no other, less intrusive means available to reach the same objective . . . restrictions must not be imposed in an arbitrary, unreasonable, or discriminatory manner.

Table 9.1 Ethical principles for communicable disease outbreaks

Ethical principle	Description
Justice	This incorporates two concepts of justice. First, equity refers to a fair distribution of resources, opportunities and outcomes. Second, procedural justice refers to a fair process for making important decisions.
Beneficence	This refers to acts that are done for the benefit of others. In a public health context, it also refers to meeting basic needs such as nourishment, shelter, health and security.
Utility	This principle states that actions are right if they promote the wellbeing of individuals or communities. These actions require consideration of proportionality and efficiency.
Respect for persons	This principle refers to treating individuals in ways informed by humanity, dignity and inherent rights. This includes autonomy, transparency and truth telling.
Liberty	Liberty includes principles that are protected as basic human rights, including freedom of movement, speech and assembly.
Reciprocity	This principle involves making a 'fitting and proportional return' for contributions that people have made.
Solidarity	This is a principle whereby groups, communities and nations stand together. Solidarity supports efforts to overcome inequalities that impact upon minorities and vulnerable populations.

Ethical codes for professions

In addition to the ethical codes and principles outlined above, many professions have ethical codes specific to that profession. The Hippocratic Oath has historically been taken by physicians as a promise to uphold ethical standards. The oath has been superseded by more contemporary codes of ethical practice, often adapted to reflect the cultures, ethics and laws of the nation or region in which the physician is practising. Organizations such as the American Medical Association, the Health Professions Council of South Africa and the UK's General Medical Council have guidelines and principles to which their practising members are expected to adhere. Other health professionals will have ethical codes that are specific and related to their fields of practice – for example, the International Council of Nurses has a Code of Ethics for Nurses.

These professional codes provide clarity and frameworks for those practising medicine or health care within those specific professions. They also provide a further dimension of ethical consideration that those professionals have to navigate: which sets of ethical principles should be prioritized if a professional is working within a setting, environment, country or institution that has competing or conflicting ethical principles to those established under ethical codes for specific professions.

Case study 9.1:   Applying ethical principles in practice

In 1999, a partnership of UK community-based HIV organizations was brought together to deliver a national HIV prevention programme for men who have sex with men (MSM) in England. Recognizing the diversity in ethos and practice in the partnership, the key organizations sought to develop a common ethical framework by which the work of the partnership would be developed. The coalition of organizations developed a model described as the 'We Decide: You Decide' axis (Bonell *et al.*, 2000). The axis was used as a way of determining who decides what people do (or do not do). In the model, 'we' was broadly seen to be authorities, institutions and bodies, and 'you' was broadly seen to be individuals and communities. At each end of the axis, the model sought to provide examples of approaches that had been previously undertaken to prevent HIV, and to determine what would, or would not, be acceptable approaches to working within the partnership. For example, 'physical intervention' refers to physically preventing an activity that might lead to HIV acquisition (such as the 'policing' of public sex environments), while 'removing barriers' refers to activity that removes obstacles to HIV prevention (such as removing bans on provision of condoms in environments where sex is occurring, such as prisons, for example):

'We Decide'	*'You Decide'*
Physical intervention	Removing barriers
Misinformation	Education
Limiting opportunity	Awareness raising
Instruction giving	Skills development
Banning	Empowerment

Adapted from Bonell *et al.* (2000)

This approach developed across the 15 years that the partnership worked together, and was an approach that was adapted and borrowed for other health conditions. The coalition used an evidenced-based approach, as well as an ethics-based approach, to inform their framework, determining that even if some unethical approaches were seen to be acceptable by some (such as the removal of autonomy in sex and sexuality), such approaches would likely be unrealistic or unenforceable.

The framework determined that acceptable approaches to HIV prevention were those on the right of the table above, and that approaches on the left would not be undertaken, supported or resourced through the partnership.

Discussion surrounding the model highlights an obvious tension: it is not the nature of an institution that determines whether it will use a more authoritarian or less authoritarian approach. It is possible that community-based organizations, for example, can impose authoritarian approaches upon its community members, or that individuals can determine that they have the right to impose any of the 'We Decide' approaches on others.

Activity 9.1

Think of some examples of decisions that policy-makers and public health practitioners make and the ethical considerations they involve. What ethical basis might these decisions be drawn from?

Feedback

Public health practitioners and policy-makers have to weigh up ethical considerations when making decisions on a regular basis, regardless of whether they consider them to be ethical issues or not. For example, decisions have to be made about whom to provide drugs or health services to in resource-poor settings. A ministry of health might decide to provide a vaccination to one population group but not to another population group because it is not deemed cost-effective to vaccinate everyone. A health adviser might have to weigh up the pros and cons of telling the close contacts of a patient that they might have been exposed to a communicable disease, at the risk of identifying the patient who may have transmitted the disease. A health authority might have to decide whether to quarantine an individual, or restrict the movement or activities of individuals in the event of an outbreak. In some instances, public health officials might enforce a treatment or vaccination of a patient, against their own wishes or beliefs, or against those of their family. In each circumstance, the decisions on how to apply an ethical framework to public health, and to communicable disease control in particular, will be informed by the ethical guidelines and principles used in their own country and organizations. In addition, their own professional ethical codes, such as the Hippocratic Oath for doctors, will play a role.

Fear and resistance

As discussed in Chapter 8, public health professionals have a role in ensuring that communication around communicable disease control does not instil fear within a population. Fear can cause officials to make poor decisions and cause individuals to act in counterproductive ways. Especially in the context of an outbreak, it is not uncommon for professionals to be working with significant levels of uncertainty, rapidly developing and escalating situations and widespread media reporting which is not always accurate. It is not uncommon for fear to spread in such circumstances. However, fear is not productive and it can be damaging to communicable disease control efforts. Fear can lead to targeting and stigmatization of vulnerable or marginalized populations. It can lead to poor decisions being made, including those that disregard ethical principles. It can generate confusion and misinformation among affected populations.

Case study 9.2: Ebola outbreak and fear

Hofman and Au (2017), reflecting on the experience of non-governmental organization (NGO) Médecins Sans Frontières (MSF) in the 2014 Ebola virus disease (EVD) outbreaks in Guinea, Liberia and Sierra Leone, state that 'fear was the catchword of this epidemic'. They write that while fear was a response to the uncertain situation involving a substantial health emergency, some of the fear was driven for political gain. Fear drove responses within West Africa and internationally, including the inflow of aid from rich donor countries. They also describe how 'noncontextualized public health messages . . . such as "Ebola kills"' resulted in individuals failing to seek treatment, assuming that seeking treatment would not assist them. The authors identify different stages of fear in the EVD epidemics, starting with those who were initially left to deal with illness and death without support from international organizations or from their local health services, which were generally inadequate even before the epidemic. Because of the transmission of EVD through intimate contact, and especially to caregivers, medics and those dealing with dead bodies, fear around social contact started to escalate. This fear was fuelled further by misinformation and uncertainty. Another stage of fear was driven by quarantine of suspected and confirmed EVD cases. Hofman and Au argue that quarantine was medical but it was also political in the sense that it demonstrated that the authorities were 'doing something'. In some instances, quarantine processes were heavy-handed, resulting in communities responding with violence and resistance to coercive powers.

A further dimension of fear was 'fear from a distance', with attempts by international players to contain the epidemic of EVD at its source. This included security measures put in place at international borders, cancellation of flights to and from West Africa, compulsory screening of travellers (often undertaken haphazardly and inadequately, arguably a further measure by authorities to demonstrate that something was being done to protect their population) and quarantining of humanitarian workers. Fears of 'contagion' spreading across the world led to disproportionate concerns that EVD was a global health threat. This global hysteria resulted in discrimination against people of African origin in Asia, Europe and North America.

Responding to fear in communicable disease control

The EVD epidemic in West Africa demonstrates the danger that information and interventions can generate fear, which is counterproductive to communicable disease control efforts. In addition to the communication guidance given in Chapter 8, communicable disease specialists need to be able to weigh up the immediate and the long-term consequences of undertaking actions that may restrict the rights of individuals or populations or be perceived as doing so. Interventions to contain or restrict the movement of populations might lead to them going underground, making them harder to reach. In addition, using the military or police to assist in a communicable disease outbreak will be highly controversial with populations that might have faced military violence or oppression. Decisions made by governments and health organizations during outbreaks may negatively impact on populations' trust of health professionals and services after the outbreak.

Summary

This chapter has introduced a range of commonly used principles of ethics, including those developed for public health and communicable disease control. It has described how those principles are used and applied in practice, and highlighted some of the tensions that arise when attempting to apply ethical principles in practice, especially in outbreak settings. Finally, the chapter has explored how fear can drive responses to communicable disease, and how fear-driven responses can lead to resistance from affected populations, which have the potential to undermine communicable disease control.

Further reading

Childress, J.F., Faden, R.R., Gaare, R.D., Gostin, L.O., Kahn, J., Bonnie, R.J. *et al.* (2002) Public health ethics: mapping the terrain, *Journal of Law, Medicine and Ethics*, 30: 170–178.

Mann, J.M., Gostin, L., Gruskin, S., Brennan, T., Lazzarini, Z. and Fineberg, H.V. (1994) Health and human rights. *Health and Human Rights*, 1: 6–23.

Selgelid, M.J. (2005) Ethics and infectious disease, *Bioethics*, 19: 272–289.

Tännsjö, T. (2013) *Understanding Ethics*. Edinburgh: Edinburgh University Press.

References

Beauchamp, T.L. and Childress, J.F. (1989) *Principles of Biomedical Ethics*. Oxford: Oxford University Press.

Bonell, C., Hickson, F., Hartley, M., Keogh, P. and Weatherburn, W. (2000) *By any means necessary? Reflecting on how HIV prevention interventions work and the changes they bring about*, Briefing paper. London: Sigma Research. Available at: https://researchonline.lshtm.ac.uk/1386880/1/report2000d.pdf.

Hofman, A. and Au, S. (2017) Introduction, in A. Hofman and S. Au (eds.) *The Politics of Fear – Médicins Sans Frontières and the West African Ebola Epidemic*. Oxford: Oxford University Press.

Schröder-Bäck, P., Duncan, P., Sherlaw, W., Brall, C. and Czabanowska, K. (2014) Teaching seven principles for public health ethics: towards a curriculum for a short course on ethics in public health programmes, *BMA Medical Ethics*, 15: 73.

World Health Organization (WHO) (2016) *Guidance for managing ethical issues in infectious disease outbreaks*. Geneva: WHO. Available at: http://apps.who.int/iris/handle/10665/250580.

10

Health systems and communicable disease control

Samuel Boland

Overview

This chapter describes health systems, highly complex structures that exist both formally and informally, and the crucial role they play in communicable disease control. The chapter begins with a definition of health systems and explains health system actors. It goes on to describe different types of health system and models of health care, including resource availability and evidence-based practice (EBP). The chapter explores how attention to health system capacity and resilience has increased following the epidemic of Ebola virus disease (EVD) in West Africa in 2014 to 2016. The chapter concludes by exploring trends in health systems, including the role of international organizations, the private sector and non-profit organizations, competing priorities and diminishing funding, the increased privatization of health systems, and increased information sharing between agencies involved in healthcare delivery.

Learning objectives

After reading this chapter, you will be able to:

- understand what a health system is, including its components and what may influence its structure and capacity
- explain competing priorities within health systems and why these can cause disagreement
- define key terms such as stewardship, service delivery, EBP and healthcare-associated infections (HCAIs)
- compare health system(s) in your own country with those of elsewhere

Key terms

Health system: The actors and institutions involved formally and informally at all levels of delivering healthcare and public health services, including health surveillance, disease prevention and health promotion, to a particular population.

Health information system: The structure and flow of how health information is shared between people, agencies and groups within a health system.

Reactivity and proactivity: The capacity to respond to and pre-empt health needs among a particular population, respectively.

Resilience: The capacity of a health system to respond to a major public health emergency, while maintaining normal service delivery.

Service delivery: The 'output' of any health system, which is the delivery of health services to a particular individual or population.

Stewardship: The governmental activity of directing competing priorities towards national health system interests.

Definition of a health system

A health system is the broad collection of individuals, institutions and financing structures that constitute the delivery of health care to a particular population. This means more than just hospitals and clinicians – in addition to service delivery, the World Health Organization (WHO) lists leadership and governance, health information systems, health financing, human resources for health, and essential medical products and technologies as fundamental components of a health system (WHO, 2010). The WHO states that a functional health system also includes 'a reliable supply of medicines and technologies, backed by adequate funding, strong health plans, and evidence-based policies' (WHO, 2017b). In addition to patient care delivered in healthcare structures such as hospitals and health centres, this could include care within the home, health promotion and educational programmes, workplace safety measures, and other public health measures and structures.

What a health system looks like differs significantly between regions and countries. The UK National Health Service (NHS) is a good example of an integrated health system, with healthcare providers integrated within a single national system financed and directed by the national government. The USA, on the other hand, has a decentralized health system made up of many independent healthcare providers, which is financed largely through private health insurance. However, all health systems are generally organized into levels of care, from the most advanced and specialized quaternary care through to family care. It is important to note that while this hierarchy is generally recognized, not all health systems have all levels of care. For example, many poorer countries do not offer quaternary care.

Some forms of care are not easily categorized. Ambulatory care (also known as outpatient care), for example, might be provided at various health system levels. Additionally, all of these services may integrate with a wider network of social care institutions, such as nursing homes and hospices.

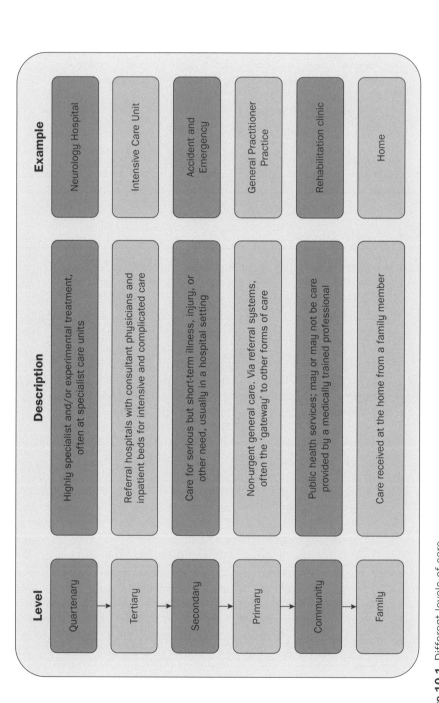

Level	Description	Example
Quarternary	Highly specialist and/or experimental treatment, often at specialist care units	Neurology Hospital
Tertiary	Referral hospitals with consultant physicians and inpatient beds for intensive and complicated care	Intensive Care Unit
Secondary	Care for serious but short-term illness, injury, or other need, usually in a hospital setting	Accident and Emergency
Primary	Non-urgent general care. Via referral systems, often the 'gateway' to other forms of care	General Practitioner Practice
Community	Public health services; may or may not be care provided by a medically trained professional	Rehabilitation clinic
Family	Care received at the home from a family member	Home

Figure 10.1 Different levels of care

Whatever the structure, it is important to remember that a health system includes everything involved in the delivery of healthcare and public health services from the home to the hospital, including the management, financing and infrastructure, which may not be visible to the user or observer.

Health system actors and influences

Politics

Politics play an important role in shaping any health system and have a significant effect. The majority of people consider health care to be an important service and good health to be a highly prioritized goal, so the politics of health systems can be powerfully ideological. There are many questions over who ultimately holds responsibility for the provision of care. Is it the responsibility of the government to provide healthcare services, as most European states contend, or should private citizens be responsible for arranging their own care with independent providers, as in the USA? To what extent are individuals responsible, and thus to what extent should individuals be accountable, for their poor health outcomes? Should the focus of a health system be on maximizing treatment availability and patient choice, or on health equity and equal access? Who holds responsibility for answering questions of medical ethics, and how should care be distributed when resources are limited? While these political questions may seem abstract and philosophical, they have serious implications for health system structure and the resulting care available to all people.

Stewardship

The WHO defines health system stewardship as 'the wide range of functions carried out by governments as they seek to achieve national health policy directives', which includes 'maintaining the strategic direction of policy development and implementation, detecting and correcting undesirable trends and distortions, articulating the case for health in national development, regulating the behaviour of a wide range of actors from healthcare financiers to healthcare providers, and establishing effective accountability mechanisms' (WHO, 2017c). The quality and success of stewardship thus depends on a government's strength relative to competing interests from other governments and the private sector, who might seek to distort or change a government's health system strategy. The need for effective stewardship is therefore acute in poorer countries reliant on development assistance, as they may be more susceptible to external government and private sector interests. Unfortunately, governments that require significant external assistance are often those least able to provide effective stewardship. In these cases, intergovernmental organizations (IGOs) like the WHO serve, in part, to advocate for and bolster this stewardship.

Service delivery

Health service delivery is the 'front end' of any health system. However, this service provision is not the only activity of a health system: health service delivery requires law, bureaucracy, institutions and funding mechanisms to effectively interface. Even within a hospital, where the primary purpose is health service delivery, a large number of staff are not clinicians but administrators, accountants and other support staff. However, all these other staff, and all this other activity which occurs within health service delivery has, as its ultimate aim, meeting patient needs whether this is by doctors and nurses caring for patients in a hospital, a non-governmental organization (NGO) providing vaccines in a school, or an IGO like the World Food Programme providing nutritional programming to the population of a refugee camp. Health service delivery is thus provided by any number of actors in any number of places – which actors, in which place and with what money is the focus of intense debate the world over.

Non-health system actors

A number of actors interact with and influence health systems but can still be considered non-health system actors if their primary role and responsibility is not, in itself, directly within the health system. One example is the military, whose primary role and responsibility is not to provide health services. However, militaries nonetheless interact with health systems, for example by providing logistics and other response support in a humanitarian emergency. Other security forces like border control provide population health monitoring, while police officers and firefighters may provide first-responder aid. Non-health system actors may not even provide health services: lawyers and legal firms may litigate cases of medical malpractice or legal frameworks surrounding health systems, while banks may provide loans to patients in need of funds for an operation. Other non-health system actors include institutions that provide health services and health education, secondary to their general purpose. This might include schools and prisons, or even workplaces that encourage employees to eat well and bicycle to work.

Potentially competing interests

A number of non-health system interests influence health systems. These interests and influences frequently surround questions of finance. The health sector is an enormous industry, accounting for an average of 10% of a country's gross domestic product (GDP) (WHO, 2014). In some countries, that figure is even higher – the USA's health spending as a proportion of GDP is 17.8%, or US$3.2 trillion annually (Centers for Medicare and Medicaid Services, 2016). The enormity of this capital flow and related profit-making enterprise inevitably attracts private sector interests, those with potentially little interest in the health system or health system delivery itself. Alternately, actors outside a health system may seek some of the money apportioned for health systems – if less money is spent by a government on health care, there is more to spend elsewhere. Philosophical disagreements also influence health systems. For example, religious arguments against the provision of contraception and abortion services can influence the availability of funding for these health services. Ideological views held by governing parties about the role of the state may influence the funding and service delivery structure of a health system.

Service recipients

Service recipients or service users are those who receive health services delivered by a health system. This may include patients receiving emergency care in a hospital, or children seeing their paediatrician for an annual check-up. However, service recipients may also be groups of people. For example, a hospital's community outreach programme may define its intended service recipients as all pre-school-aged children within a geographic area with moderate to acute malnutrition. While those that receive care are ultimately individuals, the structure of a programme may thus target entire groups of people. Here, each specific individual and the group of individuals may both be understood to be service recipients. In some cases, people who benefit from health services may include family and community members, as well as service recipients themselves. For example, health services that support pregnant women may provide secondary benefit to their existing children, or tertiary benefit to their community.

Health systems and health care

Resource availability

While health systems all aim to achieve the same basic end, the resources available to them vary significantly across the world. The WHO estimates that annual per-capita health expenditure ranges from US$9403 in the USA to just $25 in the Central African Republic (2014 estimates, 2011 PPP dollars; Centers for Medicare and Medicaid Services, 2016). This incredible diversity is also reflected in the array of funding sources. State health systems like the NHS in the UK primarily rely on government funds generated through taxation. Contrast this with the USA's privatized health service delivery, which often relies instead on private health insurance, purchased electively by each individual resident. Many countries, especially those in the Global South, also rely on bilateral aid, loans from international organizations like the World Bank, and private donations, with funds distributed to both governmental and non-governmental institutions for service delivery. Differences in resource availability can result in differences in service delivery – preventative and primary care, for example, are relatively cheap, and actors may be necessarily predisposed to promote these alternatives in lieu of more expensive treatment options.

Evidence-based practice

Evidence-based practice (EBP) seeks to standardize the delivery of patient care using methods that have been demonstrated to be effective through research. It includes evidence-based medicine (EBM), empirically supported treatments (ESTs) and evidence-based behavioural practice (EBBP). Over the past 20 years, EBP has become increasingly accepted as the 'gold standard' of clinical practice, and today dominates the design of patient care, particularly in the Global North where new research and technologies are more accessible (Thomas and Pring, 2004; Fernandez et al., 2015). While it may seem intuitive that patient care methodology should be scientifically supported, the introduction of EBP to new care centres, hospitals or health systems can be challenging. Many clinicians reject some EBPs in favour of clinical practices grounded in personal experience (Timmermans and Mauck, 2005). Indeed, some criticize EBP for oversimplifying necessarily complex problems, instead arguing that the nuances of individual patients and individual patient need – socio-economic status, family conditions and history, cultural contexts, and so forth – demand ungeneralizable and unique resolutions to individual patient care (Fernandez et al., 2015).

Healthcare-associated infections

Health systems can sometimes facilitate the propagation of the very infectious diseases they aim to treat. When an infection occurs within the hospital setting, it is known as a healthcare-associated infection HCAI, which is also sometimes referred to as a nosocomial infection. The disease burden of these nosocomial infections should not be underestimated. For example, the Centers for Disease Control and Prevention (CDC) in the USA estimate that 5–10% of all hospital admissions are due to nosocomial infections, which in 2011 resulted in 75,000 deaths (Magill et al., 2014). Much can be done to help prevent these infections, including the use of personal protective equipment by clinical staff interacting with infectious patients, the effective sterilization of surgical tools between operations, and the regular replacement of wound dressings and intravenous catheters. However, many nosocomial infections can be prevented through measures as simple and cheap as clinicians washing hands between patients and after exposure to contagious agents – although a study in the 1990s found that clinicians in the UK did do this as little as 30% of the time (Gould *et al.*, 1996). HCAIs are discussed in more detail in Chapter 6.

Supervised infectious disease therapy

As explained in Section 2, infectious diseases often require sustained drug treatment for their effective control. In the case of non-resistant bacterial infection, this may only mean a few days of antibiotic treatment. In the case of antiretroviral therapy for HIV, this means a lifetime of daily medication. Due to the risks associated with nosocomial infection, the expense of inpatient care, and the desire to provide normalcy where possible to a patient's life, sustained therapy is often provided outside the clinical setting. However, there are risks associated with unsupervised treatment, primarily surrounding lack of adherence to a prescribed drug regimen. This may not only harm a patient due to the inefficient or unsuccessful treatment of their infection, but can also drive the emergence and spread of antimicrobial resistance among infectious agents. One solution to this problem is to supervise infectious disease therapy, which is essentially the process of monitoring and ensuring the consistency of drug therapy adherence. For example, Directly Observed Treatment, Short-Course (DOTS) is the WHO's recommended strategy for the control and treatment of tuberculosis TB, and involves a community health worker monitoring drug therapy daily for two months, followed by regular check-ins with the TB patient for the remainder of the 6- to 9-month drug therapy course.

Health systems and public health

This section looks at health systems as they relate to public health and the delivery of public health services, as opposed to clinical care. Where discussed, 'public health needs' can be understood as the non-clinical health needs of a population. Public health delivery is thus generally targeted at improving population health, rather than the health of specific patients.

Resource availability

Resources for health systems are available from a variety of sources, both public and private. How much resource is required, and the source of the funding, depends on a health system's financing model. A fee-for-service (FFS) model, like that in the USA and Japan, charges for each service provided. Bundled payment, capitation and all-payer rate setting are models that attempt to discourage the over-treatment incentivized by (and therefore expense incurred by) FFS models. Whatever the health system financing model – these are several among many – health services may be compensated through one or a combination of sources, whether by the patient using personal funds, the government using funds raised through taxation, or through a public or private insurer. Other important resources available to health systems include philanthropic donations from private individuals or charitable agencies like the Bill & Melinda Gates Foundation, bilateral aid from one government to another, government grants to NGOs supporting health services, and intergovernmental loans from agencies like the World Bank and International Monetary Fund (IMF).

Surveillance and health information systems

Health surveillance is an important public health function. Chapter 4 describes different types of health surveillance and the important role it plays in communicable disease control. Communicable disease surveillance is the process of collecting, aggregating and analysing data related to disease, with the intention of quickly identifying, responding to and controlling a disease outbreak. Health surveillance data moves within a health information system, which exists as part of a health system in both formal and informal ways.

Population health

Population health is the degree of 'physical, mental, and social-wellbeing' (WHO, 2017a), not of individuals, but of a defined group of individuals as well as 'the distribution of such outcomes within the group' (Kindig and Stoddart, 2003). How populations are grouped can vary: it may be by age, ethnicity, gender, class, nationality, or just about any other metric. How health is measured among each group is similarly diverse, but is usually measured using various health indicators of quantifiable measures of health outcomes within a population. As such, population health is often used as a rough measure for comparing health systems, by looking at how the health indicators compare between one country and another, for example. It is also a powerful tool for comparing various populations within one health system, for example, by looking at how health outcomes differ by income or gender. In addition to the statistical utility of population health metrics, population health provides a powerful tool for public health targeting: a country may decide it wishes to improve childhood health, or maternal health, or sexual health among teenagers. These categorizations provide focus for health system and public health planning.

Public health response

Public health response is the response of public health actors and institutions to a public health need. How a health system develops a public health response is dependent on both the health system and public health need in question, and is thus highly circumstantial. If the public health need is acute and threatens global consequences, as was seen in the 2014–2016 West Africa Ebola epidemic, a public health response could manifest as a multifaceted, international and inter-organizational public health response, complete with extraordinary and temporary organizational structures designed to respond to the particular public health need. However, a public health response could also occur in response to more protracted, everyday problems, like the provision of health messaging in school cafeterias to help respond to the world's childhood obesity epidemic. Many countries establish specific agencies to manage public health responses, including the Centers for Disease Control and Prevention (CDC) in the USA, the China CDC, and Public Health England in England, UK. In 2017, the African Union agreed to establish the Africa Centres for Disease Control and Prevention.

✎ Activity 10.1

Think of a health system public health response to any communicable disease issue in your own community or country. Consider and articulate as many different actors and institutions involved in alleviating this particular public health need as you can, across prevention, advocacy, education and treatment spaces. What are the methods each of these actors and institutions use to do so? Where do you think the funding for this work comes from? What are the ways that these actors and institutions do and do not work together?

Feedback

You may have considered the response to a communicable disease like HIV, influenza or measles. You will have thought about the hospitals and clinicians that care for whatever health need you considered. You may have also thought about the NGOs' running billboards and televised public service announcements drawing attention to your particular issue, and the private companies encouraging individuals to seek care for it – for example, a pharmacy asking all customers whether they had received their annual flu vaccination. Some things you might have considered may not be visible – for example, the discussions and arrangements made between pharmaceutical companies and a hospital or pharmacy. You may have considered whether the hospitals near you are public or private, and what that means for their sources of available funding, as well as the private sources of funding based on private interest in the health need you considered.

Health systems trends

Increasing focus on health system resilience

The capacity of a health system to deal with emergencies is called health system resilience and varies greatly between settings. If a health system has no resilience, an emergency or the health needs resulting from it will cause health service delivery to shut down in entirety. If a health system has perfect resilience, an emergency causes no change: not only are the health needs resulting from the emergency sufficiently managed, but normal health service delivery continues as well. No health system has no resilience, and no health system has perfect resilience. Every health system has resilience somewhere between these two extremes, and may be more or less resilient to different scales and types of emergencies. This degree of resilience defines how much external support a health system requires to respond to an emergency, while maintaining core services.

Health systems research and policy are increasingly focused on the need to create health system resilience, especially following the 2014–2016 EVD epidemic.

 Activity 10.2

Read the case study below and then consider the following. What factors led to the collapse of Sierra Leone's health system during the 2014–2016 West Africa Ebola epidemic? What factors over the last 50 years led to this collapse? What could have been done to prevent this collapse? What could have been in place to contain the outbreak more quickly? What could be done now to make Sierra Leone's health system more resilient to future outbreaks?

Case study 10.1: Sierra Leone during the 2014–2016 West Africa Ebola epidemic

The capacity of a health system to deal with an emergency depends on an enormous number of factors and has significant implications for health service delivery, something the failure of Sierra Leone's health system during the 2014–2016 West Africa Ebola epidemic shows clearly. Shortly after the first cases of Ebola arrived in Sierra Leone, the WHO was notified as required by the International Health Regulations (IHR) – however, they did not immediately declare a Public Health Emergency of

International Concern (PHEIC), a declaration that facilitates external support and funding in the event of a health crisis. As such, for the first months of the Ebola outbreak, Sierra Leone's health system carried the entire burden of the outbreak more or less unsupported. Given the virulence of Ebola and the specialist facilities and equipment needed to safely care for it (which Sierra Leone did not have), many clinicians acquired the infection and died. Other clinical staff refused to come to work owing to this risk. Many hospitals and care centres therefore closed, or stopped providing some or all of the non-Ebola clinical services so desperately needed by Sierra Leoneans. Where hospitals and care centres did remain open, many patients in need stayed away, either for fear of contracting Ebola or of being sent to Ebola treatment centres. Patients with non-Ebola needs like malaria, acute diarrhoea or giving birth now went untreated and unsupported. Morbidity and mortality sky-rocketed (Cheng, 2015; Streifel, 2015; Brolin Ribacke et al., 2016).

Feedback

You may have considered a number of factors that led to the collapse of Sierra Leone's health system in the wake of the Ebola outbreak. This might have included the poor state of infection control in Sierra Leone's hospitals, their lack of human resources, or the lethargy and the complexity of international intervention. You may have also considered some 'big picture' historical questions, such as how colonialism extracted wealth from the country that could have been used to create a resilient health system, or how structural adjustment programmes in the past half century reduced governmental capacity to build new hospitals and train new staff. To help prevent the outbreak, you may have suggested external sources of funding and other resources to strengthen the country's health systems, or public health education campaigns aimed at reducing behaviours that spread communicable diseases. You may have also critiqued the international political economy that greatly influences the way money is distributed among countries and people, and suggested ways it could be adapted or changed to better resource Sierra Leone's health system.

The role of intergovernmental organizations versus for- and non-profit organizations

The main IGO concerned with health and health systems is the WHO, a constituent body of the United Nations (UN). The WHO describes its role as to support countries by 'providing leadership on matters critical to

health . . ., shaping the research agenda . . ., setting norms and standards
. . ., articulating ethical and evidence-based policy options . . ., providing
technical support . . ., [and] monitoring the health situation and assessing
health trends' (WHO, 2017d). You will note that health service delivery – in
other words, the operational activity of a health system – is not among
these responsibilities. This is accomplished through either public or private
actors, the latter divided between non-profit and for-profit providers.
For-profit providers charge for their services with the intention of creating
profit. Non-profit organizations like NGOs and philanthropic organizations,
on the other hand, are generally less concerned with financial return,
providing services that are funded not by charging users, but from government and private charitable donations. Over the last three decades, NGOs
as health service delivery mechanisms in particular have rapidly gained
power and influence, which increasingly challenges accountability and
governance recommendations maintained by the WHO (McGann and
Johnstone, 2005; Obiyan, 2005; Turner, 2010).

Competing priorities and diminishing funding

Wherever resources are limited, prioritization of funding will occur: health
priorities are weighed not in relation to their intrinsic merit, but by their
relative significance to other health priorities. Low- and middle-income
countries must often decide whether available funding goes towards paediatric care, malaria prevention, nutritional programming, or any of the other
hundreds of health needs that present. Decisions must also be made
whether to prioritize support to tertiary and urban care centres versus rural
and peripheral care centres, and how to weigh resources between preventative and curative care. Even in relatively well-funded health systems like
the NHS in the UK, decisions are made about whether high-cost treatments
should be provided with limited government funds when more cost-efficient
but potentially less efficacious alternatives exist (Macmillan and Cancerbackup, 2011). Particularly in the face of fiscal crisis and subsequent
austerity measures like those seen after the economic recession of the
late 2000s, the implications of this competition grow stronger and the
negative consequences for patient care greater (Karanikolos et al., 2013).

Increasing privatization

Through the 1950s, health service delivery was increasingly realized
through the state – as states became stronger and better resourced, state-
funded and state-provided health services followed (Blanchette and Tolley,
2001). However, with increasing globalization in the second half of the
twentieth century, markets became an increasingly popular tool for measur-
ing and guiding public policy, grounded in the liberal economic philosophy
favoured in the USA and the West. When not adopted, this philosophy was

sometimes enforced: beginning in the 1950s, conditional loans to low- and middle-income countries from the World Bank and IMF mandated structural adjustment programs (SAPs). These SAPs required liberal economic restructuring, which resulted in the withdrawal of the state from health service delivery in favour of private sector or public–private alternatives. Particularly in the Global South, this shift to market-driven health service delivery can be seen in the proliferation of NGOs, which fill some health service delivery gaps previously addressed by the state (Turner, 2010). The debate about the role of the state in providing and financing health care continues today, with some arguing that the state has a responsibility to ensure health service delivery and equity of access, and others arguing that individuals should have responsibility for and control over their own health and health care.

✎ **Activity 10.3**

Consider your own health system(s). In what ways are your health services delivered by the state, and in what ways are they delivered by the private sector? Try and be as comprehensive as possible – maybe your health system utilizes government hospitals, but medical education and peripheral services are provided by private sector organizations. Are you aware of any current conversations and debates related to increased privatization in your health system(s)?

Feedback

Depending on where you live and where you are from, your answers to these questions will vary significantly. You will have thought about the hospitals around you, and whether those are run by a national health service, or by a university or company. You will have thought about whether patients are expected to pay for any health services they receive – even within a national health service, some things (prescriptions, transport, elective procedures, etc.) do cost patients money. You may also have thought about some NGOs that provide specific health services, like access to abortion and contraceptive services.

Reactive versus proactive systems

Health systems are both reactive and proactive, and all health care exists on a spectrum between the two. A reactive health system component responds to health needs as they present. For example, a hospital reacts to sickness among its patients by providing curative treatment or palliative care. A proactive health system component, on the other hand, anticipates and addresses the causes of health needs before they arise. Primary and public health measures, including nutritional programmes, educational outreach and even poverty alleviation are good examples of proactive health system components. The two are inextricably linked – a doctor providing reactive treatment may also provide proactive health education to their patient, for example. However, different philosophies of care and different funding priorities may result in the balance shifting more towards one than the other. Preventative care is generally cheaper and less technologically demanding than reactive care, and is thus of huge importance in terms of cost-efficiency. Reactive health systems, on the other hand, may be more expensive, but are nonetheless a crucial part of a health system whole: no amount of proactive work can prevent all need for reactivity.

Technological developments in health care and healthcare expenditure

Adjusted for inflation, healthcare expenditure per capita is increasing in most of the world's nations (Kaiser Family Foundation, 2011). Much of this is due to an increased focus on the importance of health care, while other key factors include technological developments in health care and the broader shift in some nations to specialist and highly technical medical care. For example, improvements in intensive and critical care result in improvements to health outcomes (Luce and Rubenfeld, 2002). However, intensive and critical care are extremely expensive and represent an increasingly large fraction of health care and thus healthcare expenditure (Luce and Rubenfeld, 2002).

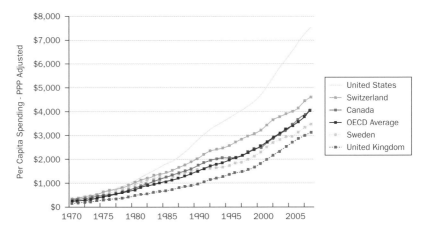

Figure 10.2 Per capita healthcare spending over time

Source: Kaiser Family Foundation (2011).

While increased healthcare expenditure per capita generally correlates with improvements in most health indices, this is not always the case. The biggest exception to this correlation is in the USA, for which per capita healthcare costs exceed the next highest spender by 50%. For example, the WHO ranks the USA as 31st in life expectancy at birth and 30th for under-five mortality (Kaiser Family Foundation, 2011; WHO, 2015, 2016). Some argue this is the result of a for-profit system focusing too heavily on expensive and therefore profitable technological interventions, rather than non-profit nationalized systems that benefit from cost-control measures and therefore focus more heavily on public health interventions (Sullivan, 2016).

Increased information sharing

Because the care of any one patient or population is usually shared between many actors, information sharing within a health information system is a crucial component of any health system. However, this information sharing is less than straightforward, often precisely because of this multitude of health service providers, with many actors requiring access to patient data created across multiple sites. Some of the challenges to information sharing are simply logistical: many low-income countries do not have the infrastructure for electronic records, and paper records are notoriously difficult to manage appropriately and efficiently. Even in high-income countries, however, technical challenges to information sharing abound. The electronic medical record (EMR) (alternatively 'electronic patient record' or EPR) business is a multibillion dollar industry, yet even those considered among the most cutting-edge and sought after are replete with implementation failures and difficulties. For example, the NHS in the UK recently spent £200 million piloting a new EMR that immediately resulted in widespread difficulties (Bawden, 2014). Finally, some challenges to information sharing are philosophical: patient information is generally considered confidential, so legally sharing health data, even with patient consent and the technical capacity to do so, can be challenging.

Summary

Health systems play a central role in communicable disease control. The scale of human need for health service delivery is enormous and health systems help provide it, from a parent caring for their sick child at home to a multibillion dollar network of hospitals. Health service delivery requires substantial resources and health systems are highly complex. Consequently, there are different approaches to financing, structuring and delivering health services. Disagreements often arise over questions of funding and prioritization amid scarce and diminishing resources. A wide range of interests and influences shape health systems. Recent trends include privatization of health services and an increased role for non-profit organizations. There are also concerns about cost-efficiency as more technologically advanced and expensive treatments become available. Debates about rights and responsibilities of the state and individuals in health and health care continue, with consequences for health systems, health care and health outcomes.

References

Bawden, J. (2014) *Recent pressures in the Cambridge and South Cambridgeshire health system*. Cambridge: Cambridgeshire and Peterborough Clinical Commissioning Group. https://ehrintelligence.com/images/site/articles/2014-12-01-Recent-Pressures-in-the-Cambridge-and-South-Cambridgeshire.pdf

Blanchette, C. and Tolley, E. (2001) *Public- and Private-Sector Involvement in Health-Care Systems: A Comparison of OECD Countries*. Ottawa: Government of Canada.

Brolin Ribacke, K.J., van Duinen, A., Nordenstedt, H., Höijer, J., Molnes, R., Froseth, T.W. *et al*. (2016) The impact of the West Africa Ebola outbreak on obstetric health care in Sierra Leone, *PLoS ONE*, 11: (2). doi: 10.1371/journal.pone.0150080.

Centers for Medicare and Medicaid Services (2016) *Historical National Health Expenditure Accounts (NHEA)*. Centers for Medicaire & Medicaid Services. December 6. https://www.cms.gov/research-statistics-data-and-systems/statistics-trends-and-reports/nationalhealthexpenddata/nationalhealthaccountshistorical.html

Cheng, M. (2015) Malaria killed more people than usual in Ebola outbreak, *The Washington Times*, 23 June. Available at: http://www.washingtontimes.com/news/2015/jun/23/malaria-killed-more-people-than-usual-in-ebola-out/

Fernandez, A., Sturmberg, J., Lukersmith, S., Madden, R., Torkfar, G., Colagiuri, R. *et al*. (2015) Evidence-based medicine: is it a bridge too far?, *Health Research Policy and Systems*, 13: 66.

Gould, D., Wilson-Barnett, J. and Ream, E. (1996) Nurses' infection-control practice: hand decontamination, the use of gloves and sharp instruments, *International Journal of Nursing Studies*, 33 (2): 143–160.

Kaiser Family Foundation (2011) *Snapshots: Health care spending in the United States & selected OECD countries*, The Henry J. Kaiser Family Foundation, 12 April 2011. Available at: http://kff.org/health-costs/issue-brief/snapshots-health-care-spending-in-the-united-states-selected-oecd-countries/

Karanikolos, M., Mladovsky, P., Cylus, J., Thomson, S., Basu, S., Stuckler, D. *et al*. (2013). Financial crisis, austerity, and health in Europe, *The Lancet*, 381 (9874): 1323–1331.

Kindig, D. and Stoddart, G. (2003) What is population health?, *American Journal of Public Health*, 93 (3): 380–383.

Luce, J.M. and Rubenfeld, G. (2002) Can health care costs be reduced by limiting intensive care at the end of life?, *American Journal of Respiratory and Critical Care Medicine*, 165 (6): 750–754.

Macmillan and Cancerbackup (2011) *What you can do if a treatment is not available*. Available at: http://www.nhs.uk/ipgmedia/national/Macmillan%20Cancer%20Support/Assets/WhatyoucandoiftreatmentisntavailableMCS6pages.pdf

McGann, J. and Johnstone, M. (2005) The power shift and the NGO credibility crisis, *The Brown Journal of World Affairs*, 11 (2): 159–172.

Magill, S.S., Edwards, J.R., Beldavs, Z.G., Dumyati, G., Janelle, S.J., Kainer, M.A. *et al*. (2014) Prevalence of antimicrobial use in US acute care hospitals, May–September 2011, *Journal of the American Medical Association*, 312 (14): 1438–1446.

Obiyan, A.S. (2005) A critical examination of the state versus non-governmental organizations (NGOs) in the policy sphere in the Global South: will the state die as the NGOs thrive in Sub-Saharan Africa and Asia?, *African and Asian Studies*, 4 (3): 301–326.

Streifel, C. (2015) *How did Ebola impact maternal and child health in Liberia and Sierra Leone?* Washington, DC: Center for Strategic and International Studies. Available at: https://www.csis.org/analysis/how-did-ebola-impact-maternal-and-child-health-liberia-and-sierra-leone

Sullivan, N. (2016) Why is healthcare so expensive in the United States?, *The Hill*, 6 December. Available at: http://thehill.com/blogs/pundits-blog/healthcare/309069-why-is-healthcare-so-expensive-in-the-united-states

Thomas, G. and Pring, R. (eds.) (2004) *Evidence-Based Practice in Education*. Maidenhead: McGraw-Hill Education.

Timmermans, S. and Mauck, A. (2005) The promises and pitfalls of evidence-based medicine, *Health Affairs*, 24 (1): 18–28.

Turner, E.A.L. (2010) Why has the number of international non-governmental organizations exploded since 1960?, *Cliodynamics: The Journal of Theoretical and Mathematical History*, 1: 81–91.

World Health Organization (WHO) (2010) *Key components of a well functioning health system*. Geneva: WHO. Available at: http://www.who.int/healthsystems/publications/hss_key/en/

World Health Organization (WHO) (2014) *Global health expenditure*. Geneva: WHO.

World Health Organization (WHO) (2015) *Under-five mortality rate*. Geneva: WHO.

World Health Organization (WHO) (2016) *World health statistics 2016: Monitoring health for the SDGs*. Geneva: WHO. Available at: http://www.who.int/gho/publications/world_health_statistics/2016/en/

World Health Organization (WHO) (2017a) *Constitution of the World Health Organization*. Geneva: WHO. Available at: http://apps.who.int/gb/bd/PDF/bd47/EN/constitution-en.pdf

World Health Organization (WHO) (2017b) *Health systems*. Geneva: WHO. Available at: http://www.who.int/healthsystems/about/progress-challenges/en/

World Health Organization (WHO) (2017c) *Stewardship*. Geneva: WHO. Available at: http://www.who.int/healthsystems/stewardship/en/

World Health Organization (WHO) (2017d) *The role of WHO in public health*. Geneva: WHO. Available at: http://www.who.int/about/role/en/

11 Emerging trends, challenges and opportunities in communicable disease control

Liza Cragg

Overview

The opening chapter of this book gave a brief historical overview of the development of communicable disease control. This chapter explores emerging trends in communicable disease and the environmental, economic and social factors that are driving these trends. The chapter examines antimicrobial resistance, one of the key challenges to communicable disease control, its causes and its potential impact. It briefly explores developments in global health governance and financing and critiques of these. It finishes by outlining several developing opportunities for communicable disease control.

Learning objectives

After reading this chapter, you will be able to:

- explain how communicable diseases are changing
- describe the environmental, social and economic factors that drive these changes
- understand the causes and potential impact of antimicrobial resistance and what needs to be done to counter it
- describe emerging opportunities in communicable disease control

Key terms

Antibiotic resistance (ABS): The ability of bacteria to protect themselves against the effects of an antibiotic.

Antimicrobial resistance (AMR): The resistance of a microorganism to an antimicrobial drug that was originally effective for treatment of infections it caused.

Emerging infectious diseases (EIDS): Infectious diseases that have appeared in a population for the first time, or that existed previously but are rapidly increasing in incidence and/or geographic range.

> **Multidrug-resistant tuberculosis (MDR-TB):** A form of tuberculosis (TB) that is resistant to treatment with at least the two most powerful anti-TB drugs (rifampicin and isoniazid).
>
> **Extensively drug-resistant tuberculosis (XDR-TB):** A form of TB that is resistant to at least four of the core anti-TB drugs.

Trends in communicable disease

Since the mid-twentieth century there have been significant changes in mortality rates and the causes of mortality, which have seen chronic and degenerative diseases become more important than communicable disease as a cause of death. This process has become known as the epidemiologic transition (Omran, 2005). Although this transition began earlier and is more pronounced in high-income countries, it is also apparent in middle-income and, increasingly, low-income countries.

As explained in Chapter 1, developments in communicable disease control led some specialists to predict that infectious diseases might become a thing of the past. However, a recent study analysing data since 1980 found that the number of outbreaks and the number of communicable diseases that cause them have actually increased over this time (Smith et al., 2014). Furthermore, as the 2014–2016 outbreak of Ebola virus disease (EVD) in West Africa demonstrated, communicable disease epidemics can cause significant mortality and have devastating social and economic costs for the countries affected.

Emerging infectious diseases (EIDs) is the term used to describe diseases that are new or reappearing. They include:

- new diseases resulting from changes in existing organisms;
- previously unknown diseases;
- known diseases spreading to new geographic areas or populations;
- old diseases re-emerging, for example as a result of antimicrobial resistance or breakdowns in public health measures (CDC, 2017).

Examples of diseases that appeared to be declining and within reach of elimination goals several decades ago but are now resurging include malaria, measles, yellow fever and TB. Examples of diseases that have been identified in the last 40 years include EVD, HIV, severe acute respiratory syndrome (SARS), hantavirus pulmonary syndrome, and influenza A/H1N1-pdm09, which caused the 2009 influenza pandemic. There is growing recognition among scientists and global health leaders that the emergence of a new infectious disease with the potential for very significant mortality is likely, or even inevitable, and more needs to be done to prepare for this (Gates, 2015; *New Scientist*, 2017).

Factors driving the emergence and spread of communicable disease

Research has identified a range of environmental, social and economic factors that contribute to the emergence of new communicable diseases and the increased spread of existing ones. These factors are not separate phenomena; indeed, they are often mutually re-enforcing and interact in dynamic ways. Many are anthropogenic factors – that is, factors originating from human activity. The ways that humans have changed land use and eco-systems have accelerated over recent decades. These include deforestation, intensified agriculture, urbanization and irrigation. A recent systematic review identified several mechanisms by which land-use change impacts on communicable disease, including changes in host and vector community composition, changes in behaviour or movement of vectors and/or hosts, altered spatial distribution of hosts and/or vectors, and environmental contamination (Gottdenker et al., 2014).

Climate change is an important anthropogenic factor that impacts on communicable disease. The survival and reproduction of vectors, pathogens and hosts are influenced by climatic conditions, including temperature, precipitation, sea level, elevation, wind and daylight duration. World Health Organization (WHO) modelling predicts that by 2030 there will be 10% more diarrhoeal disease than there would have been without climate change, and that it will primarily affect the health of young children. If global temperatures increase by 2–3°C, as expected, the number of people at risk of malaria will increase by several hundred million and the seasonal duration of malaria will increase in many currently endemic areas. It is clear from the data that developing regions of the world have been disproportionately affected by climate change compared with developed regions (Shuman, 2010).

Population growth, increasing average incomes and the emerging global-consumer class have led to a huge increase in intensive animal farming and meat production. There is evidence to suggest that intensive animal farming practices may result in fast-growing, early transmitted and more lethal pathogens because these practices differ substantially from how animals live in natural ecosystems. Whereas animals in natural ecosystems tend to exist in relatively low population densities with high immunological and ecological variation, those in intensive farms exist in higher densities of immunologically similar populations. Their diets are likely to be repetitive and may lack micronutrients, they have close contact with faeces, discarded feathers and dead animals, and may have little or no exposure to sterilizing sunlight. For example, highly pathogenic avian influenza (HPAI), which has threatened to cause a human pandemic, generally occurs and is sustained only in intensively farmed conditions (WHO, 2013). Increased trade of live animals and animal products within and between countries in recent decades also has implications for disease emergence and spread.

The urban population of the world has grown rapidly from 746 million in 1950 to 3.9 billion in 2014. As a result of this rapid urbanization, more than half the world's population lives in cities (UNDESA, 2014). Urbanization does not inevitably lead to poorer health outcomes; indeed, living conditions and access to health and other services in cities are generally better in urban environments than rural settings (Neiderud, 2015). However, very rapid and unplanned urbanization leads to the growth of slums. One-third of urban dwellers live in slums, which are characterized by extremely high population densities, overcrowded and poor quality housing, lack of sanitation, high rates of poverty and undernutrition, and changes in mobility and patterns of sexual relations. The characteristics of slums create a favourable setting for some disease vectors, animal reservoirs such as rodents, and environmental reservoirs such as contaminated water and soil. In addition, the population density of inhabitants and the close contact between people in urban areas facilitate the rapid spread of communicable disease. This means that cities can be incubators for new epidemics and the conditions to enable a worldwide pandemic could be met in urban centres (Neiderud, 2015).

Globalization can have significant impacts on the emergence, spread and control of communicable disease. Globalization describes the process of people, products and capital travelling the world in greater numbers and at greater speed, leading to increased interdependency and connectedness between countries and regions. Although globalization is not a new phenomenon, it has intensified in recent decades. The increase in frequency, speed and distance of movement of people and products enables infectious agents to move with them. Examples of the effects of globalization on the emergence, distribution and spread of communicable disease include the worldwide resurgence of dengue fever, the introduction of West Nile virus into New York City in 1999, the rapid spread of HIV infection in Russia and the global spread of MDR-TB (Knobler et al., 2006). Furthermore, the gains and losses globalization generates are unequally distributed among population groups and individuals, which has resulted in different levels of vulnerabilities to epidemics (Saker et al., 2004).

One aspect of globalization is mass migration. In 2015, 244 million people, or 3.3% of the world's population, lived outside their country of origin (UNFPA, 2017). While the majority of migrants choose to leave their countries of origin in search of better economic and social opportunities, millions of people are forced to flee due to conflict or persecution. According to the UN Refugee Agency, in 2015 over 65 million people around the world had been forced from their homes, marking the highest levels of displacement on record (UNHCR, 2016). Migrants and forced migrants are in some cases more vulnerable to communicable disease, as they may not have the immunity of the host country or region's indigenous population. In addition, migrants often come from countries affected by conflict or economic crisis and undertake long, difficult journeys that increase their own risks for communicable diseases, including measles and food and water-borne diseases. However, evidence shows the risk of a disease outbreak in a host country's population as a result of the arrival of migrants is very low (ECDC, 2015).

Finally, tackling poverty and ensuring access to services is key to pre-venting communicable diseases (Ranscombe, 2015). However, figures show that at least 400 million people still do not have access to essential health services (WHO, 2015). Lack of access to vaccination and other prevention measures, diagnostic facilities and appropriate treatment facilitates the spread of communicable disease. The global Multidimen-sional Poverty Index (MPI), which captures severe deprivation in education, health and living standards, estimates that 1.6 billion people experience poverty, of whom nearly half are destitute (OPHI, 2016). In addition to lacking access to essential health services, people living in poverty do not have access to adequate housing, sanitation, nutrition, water and other basic services, which means they are more likely to suffer and die from communicable disease.

✎ Activity 11.1

Research shows that more than 60% of emerging infectious diseases are zoonoses. This means they are diseases emerging in humans that are caused by pathogens of animal origin, and the proportion of commu-nicable diseases caused by zoonoses is increasing (Jones *et al.*, 2008). Why do you think this is?

Feedback

You might have included the following points:

- The human population has increased and expanded into new geographic areas, so more people and their domestic animals live in proximity to wild animal reservoirs. This close contact makes it easier for diseases to pass between animals and people.
- Climate change may have altered the geographic range or population dynamics of animal reservoirs and/or of vectors (such as mosquitoes) that can facilitate disease transmission between animals and humans.
- Changes in land use, such as deforestation and intensive farming practices, have impacted on the natural habitats of wild animals, in some cases causing them to live in closer proximity to humans and their livestock.
- More intensive animal farming practices create high densities of genetically homogenous livestock populations, which can amplify

> the transmission and virulence of animal pathogens that can spread to humans.
> - Urbanization and slum growth has created ideal conditions for rodents and insects that carry diseases to thrive and live in close proximity to humans.
> - Increased international trade and travel means disease can spread very quickly.
> - Increased surveillance in both human and animal populations may also have led to improved detection rates of zoonoses, which previously may not have been detected or may not have been identified as of animal origin.

The development of AMR

At the same time as outbreaks and EIDs are increasing, the availability of effective treatment for communicable disease is under threat. AMR is the resistance of a microorganism to an antimicrobial drug that was originally effective for treatment of the infections it caused. AMR includes resistance of the different types of infectious agents to the drugs that are used to treat them, including fungi, viruses, parasitic protozoans and bacteria. AMR develops when a pathogen becomes resistant to a drug so the infected person does not respond to treatment. The drug-resistant strain of the disease then spreads as the infected person passes this on to the people they infect. AMR is rapidly becoming a major public health risk. It is estimated to cause around 700,000 deaths a year and projections show this could rise to 10 million deaths a year by 2050, which would make AMR the major cause of death globally, as illustrated in Figure 11.1 (O'Neill, 2014). AMR also has a huge economic cost, both in terms of the additional healthcare and drug costs of treating individuals with infections that involve AMR microorganisms and in terms of the financial impact of additional mortality and morbidity. Furthermore, AMR threatens to undermine many of the cornerstones of modern medicine and health care. For example, many routine medical procedures would become too risky to undertake without antibiotics that work and chemotherapy for cancer, would become much more dangerous.

ABR is the form of AMR that has received most attention. It describes the ability of bacteria to protect themselves against the effects of an antibiotic. Very high rates of resistance have already been observed in bacteria that cause common healthcare-associated and community-acquired infections, including urinary tract, blood and wound infections and pneumonia. ABR is present in all countries (WHO, 2016a). There is evidence that some communicable diseases may soon become untreatable as a result of resistance to last-resort antibiotics. For example, *Neisseria gonorrhoeae* has

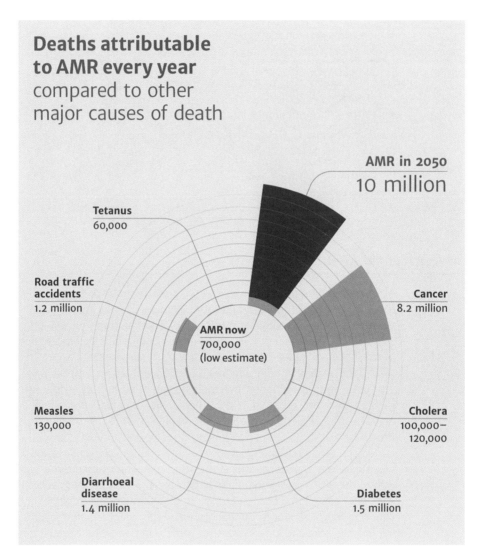

Figure 11.1 Deaths attributable to AMR versus other causes of death

Source: O'Neill (2014).

been shown to have decreased susceptibility to cephalosporins, the treatment of last resort for gonorrhoea, in 36 countries (WHO, 2014). TB is a particular concern. The WHO estimates that, in 2014, there were about 480,000 new cases of MDR-TB, a form of tuberculosis that is resistant to the two most powerful anti-TB drugs, rifampicin and isoniazid. MDR-TB requires treatment courses that are much longer and less effective than those for non-resistant TB. In 2014, only half of MDR-TB patients globally were successfully treated. XDR-TB, a form of TB that is resistant to at least four of the core anti-TB drugs, has been identified in 105 countries (WHO, 2016a).

Resistance to antiviral medications is another form of AMR. The WHO estimates that in 2010, 7% of people starting HIV antiretroviral therapy (ART) in developing countries and 10–20% in developed countries had drug-resistant HIV. The figures are even higher among people who have stopped treatment and are re-starting (WHO, 2016a). HIV drug resistance is strongly associated with increased risk for disease progression and poorer outcomes (WHO, 2014). Antiviral drugs are also important for treatment of epidemic and pandemic influenza. In 2016, the WHO reported that virtually all influenza A viruses circulating in humans were resistant to one category of antiviral drugs (M2 inhibitors), although resistance to others remains low (WHO, 2016a).

Resistance to artemisinin-based combination therapies (ACTs), which is the first-line treatment for the most dangerous form of malaria, *Plasmodium falciparum* malaria, had been confirmed in five countries by mid-2016: Cambodia, the Lao People's Democratic Republic, Myanmar, Thailand and Viet Nam. Along the Cambodia–Thailand border, *P. falciparum* has become resistant to almost all available antimalarial medicines (WHO, 2016a). This makes treatment much more expensive and difficult, resulting in poorer treatment outcomes. Given that malaria remains one of the most widespread communicable diseases, with an estimated 212 million cases a year, the potential impact of the spread of resistance to ACTs in terms of increased mortality and morbidity is enormous and threatens to reverse progress in malaria control (WHO, 2016b).

ABR occurs naturally over time as pathogens evolve to resist the new drugs that are developed to combat them. However, it has become a much more serious problem in recent years for a number of reasons. Antimicrobial use and misuse is rising. Between 2000 and 2010, consumption of antibiotic drugs increased by 36% and there was increased consumption of last-resort classes of antibiotic drugs (Van Boeckel *et al.*, 2014). A lack of understanding about the dangers of the unnecessary and improper use of antimicrobials is widespread. For example, patients often demand antibiotics from their doctors or buy them over-the-counter, even if they have a condition that antibiotics will be ineffective against. Patients also often stop taking their medications when symptoms improve, not understanding that failing to complete the entire course can lead to drug resistance. Poor practice among clinicians contributes to the problem. It is still common practice for clinicians to prescribe antibiotics based only on assessment of patient symptoms, rather than using diagnostics to ascertain what is causing the symptoms and what medication, if any, is required. Clinicians also sometimes treat with inappropriate regimens, either because treatment guidelines do not exist or because they are not used. For example, a recent study of treatment practices of TB in India, which has over a quarter of the global TB and MDR-TB burden, found 106 doctors prescribed 63 different drug regimens and only three of these 106 doctors could write an appropriate prescription for treatment of MDR-TB (Udwadia *et al.*, 2010). Inadequate application of effective communicable disease control measures, such as vaccination and good infection control, also contributes to the growth of AMR by increasing the preventable cases of disease that then require treatment with antimicrobials.

An additional factor contributing to the growth of AMR is the increasing use of antimicrobials in animal farming over the past decade, where they are used to maintain animal health, ensure growth and maximize productivity. This contributes to the spread of drug-resistant pathogens in both livestock and humans. For example, in the United States the distribution of medically important antibiotics for use in food animals increased by 26% from 2009 to 2015 (FDA, 2016). Research suggests that antimicrobial consumption will rise by 67% by 2030, as a result of increased demand for meat and the spread of intensive farming (Van Boeckel *et al.*, 2015).

Importantly, over the same period that AMR has been increasing, research into and production of new antimicrobials has slowed dramatically. In 1990, 18 pharmaceutical companies were researching antibiotics but by 2010 this had fallen to just four. Over the same 20-year period, the number of new antibiotics approved for use every year dropped significantly while resistant strains of bacteria increased markedly (Cooper and Shlaes, 2011). The commercial return for research and development of new antibiotics is not attractive for several reasons. Patients only take them for a short amount of time compared with drugs for chronic conditions. Resistance over time is inevitable, thus any antibiotic becomes less profitable. Finally, new drugs for resistant bacteria are often held in reserve by doctors to treat only the most stubborn infections, so again they are not profitable (Clarke, 2003).

AMR is a major public health emergency that is already affecting all countries in the world. However, its impact will be much greater in countries that already have high malaria, HIV or TB rates as resistance to current treatments increases. Africa as a continent will be particularly badly affected, and the impacts of HIV and TB co-morbidity already seen in many of the poorest parts of the world are likely to become worse. Figure 11.2 shows the global distribution of projected annual deaths by 2050 as a result of AMR if the problem is not addressed (O'Neill, 2014).

✎ **Activity 11.2**

What type of action do you think is necessary to stop the growth of AMR?

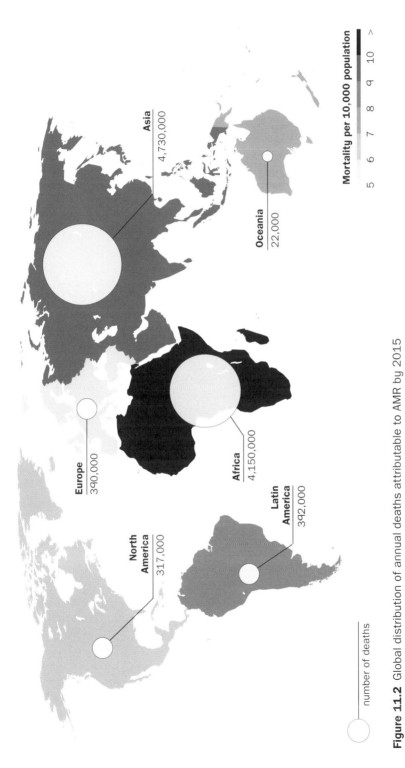

Figure 11.2 Global distribution of annual deaths attributable to AMR by 2015

Source: O'Neill (2014).

Mortality per 10,000 population

5 6 7 8 9 10 >

number of deaths

North America
317,000

Europe
390,000

Asia
4,730,000

Africa
4,150,000

Latin America
392,000

Oceania
22,000

Feedback

You might have included the following types of actions, which are taken from the *Review on Antimicrobial Resistance – Tackling drug-resistant infections globally* (O'Neill, 2016).

- A massive global public awareness campaign to improve awareness of AMR across the board, so that patients and farmers do not demand, and clinicians and veterinarians do not prescribe, antibiotics when they are not needed.
- Improve hygiene and prevent the spread of infection because the fewer people there are who get infected, the less they need to use medicines such as antibiotics, and so the less resistance to those drugs arises.
- Reduce unnecessary use of antimicrobials in agriculture and their dissemination into the environment.
- Improve global surveillance of drug resistance and antimicrobial consumption in humans and animals.
- Promote new, rapid diagnostics to cut unnecessary use of antibiotics, including making it mandatory that by 2020 the prescription of antibiotics will need to be informed by data and testing technology, wherever available and effective, in informing the doctor's judgement to prescribe.
- Promote development and use of vaccines that prevent infections and therefore lower the demand for therapeutic treatments.
- Improve the numbers, pay and recognition of people working in infectious disease because at the current time focusing on AMR-related specialties is often less rewarding financially and of less prestige than other areas of science and medicine.
- Establish a Global Innovation Fund for early-stage and non-commercial research because there is insufficient private and public investment in research and development (R&D) focused on tackling AMR.
- Provide better incentives to promote investment for new drugs and improving existing ones.
- Build a global coalition for real action, for example via the G20 and the United Nations (UN), as AMR is not a problem that can be solved by any one country, region or agency.

Developments in global health priorities and financing

Outbreaks, EIDs and AMR interact with and are influenced by other factors that shape global health priorities, including who provides funding and who exerts influence. As explained in Chapter 10, financing for public health and healthcare services varies greatly between countries. While there is a trend of increasing government expenditure on health in low- and middle-income countries and universal health coverage is increasingly recognized as a priority, in many countries health expenditure remains below required levels (IHME, 2016). Consequently, many countries in the world continue to rely on development assistance from governments in high-income countries and other donors for funding for essential health services, including communicable disease control. For example, governments of malaria-endemic countries provided 32% of total malaria funding in 2015, with the remaining 68% coming from development assistance from donors. The United States is the largest single international malaria funder and provided an estimated 35% of global funding in 2015 (WHO, 2017a). Future projections indicate that development assistance will continue to play a crucial role in supporting health systems in LMICs for many years (IHME, 2016). However, the continued provision of this essential funding is not guaranteed, as it depends on the economic and political priorities of donor governments and other providers of aid.

Over recent years, large private philanthropic organizations have become more significant contributors to development assistance for health. In particular, the Bill and Melinda Gates Foundation has emerged as a major global health player since it was set up in 1994. The Foundation's current expenditure is over US$4 billion annually. In addition to its direct funding, which has financed access to vaccinations, prevention and treatments for millions of people at risk of or suffering from infectious diseases, it has helped generate considerable global commitment to addressing health problems affecting low-income countries and poor communities. Its funding for research has also had a critical impact on international policy and thinking on infectious diseases and has provided new dynamism, credibility and attractiveness to global health issues (*The Lancet*, 2009). The trend for philanthropic foundations to become more significant funders of and players in global health looks set to continue, with the announcement in 2015 of a major philanthropic initiative, the Chan Zuckerberg Initiative, which will spend up to $40 billion (IHME, 2016).

However, large philanthropic foundations have also been challenged for their ability to exert considerable power over global policies, including health, while remaining unaccountable (Curtis, 2016). The large scale of leading philanthropic foundations' funding, which exceeds that of some UN agencies and donor governments, means they can effectively decide which issues are prioritized and which are not. Since 1990, the percentage of development assistance for health that is disbursed by UN agencies and bi-lateral agencies has decreased while the percentage disbursed by non-governmental organizations (NGOs), foundations and partnerships with the private sector has increased (IHME, 2016). In addition, some commentators have questioned the assumption that large philanthropic foundations use their funding and influence without regard to the business interests that fund them, suggesting the businesses behind the foundations often contribute to the very economic instability and inequality the foundations are supposedly seeking to solve (McGoey, 2015).

An additional aspect of health system financing relates to the investment and pricing policies of the pharmaceutical industry. There have been growing concerns over recent years about pharmaceutical companies' unfair charging policies for some medicines (Hawkes, 2016). There are also concerns about the lack of engagement and investment by major multinational pharmaceutical companies in drugs, vaccines and diagnostics for neglected tropical diseases (Hotez *et al.*, 2016). *The Lancet's* Commission on Essential Medicines Policies recently concluded that many people worldwide do not have access to even a limited basket of essential medicines. Furthermore, it found that 'the present system for developing medicines is in crisis, largely failing to produce much needed products that address the health needs of millions of people worldwide. The prices of new essential medicines that are developed are sometimes so high that even high-income countries face financing problems'. It made a range of recommendations to improve the affordability and accessibility of medicine and to develop an independent accountability system to protect investments made in essential medicines and ensure these investments translate into health and development for all (Wirtz *et al.*, 2016).

Since the 1990s, there has been increasing concern among international agencies and many governments about the potential threat to international security of infectious diseases spreading across borders or infectious agents being used in terrorist attacks, known as bioterrorism. This process has been termed the 'securitization of health'. Infectious diseases are conceptualized as security threats that require action by national and international military and security authorities, rather than public health problems. One example of this trend is the WHO's 2007 World Health Day's theme: International Health Security (WHO, 2007). Another example is UN Security Council Resolution 2177 (2014), adopted at an emergency meeting on 18 September 2014, which declared the unprecedented extent of the outbreak of Ebola virus disease in Africa a threat to international peace and security (UNSC, 2014).

However, the securitization of health has been criticized as leading to the increased politicization of aid at the expense of effective programmes, unexpected funding challenges due to geopolitical priorities, and the blurring of civilian and military institutions (Baringer and Heitkamp, 2012). There are also questions about how effective this approach is in practice. In the response to the EVD epidemic in West Africa, the international community lacked proper coordination and leadership, existing international mechanisms could not compensate for weak national health systems, and state capacities and armed forces were already stretched (Elbe and Roemer-Mahler, 2015).

Opportunities

There are also opportunities for new developments and improvements in communicable disease control. The WHO has initiated a reform process with the aim of ensuring greater coherence in global health, addressing agreed global health priorities, and ensuring the WHO's capacity to prepare for and respond to outbreaks. This has led to the WHO Health Emergencies Programme, which works with countries and partners to prepare for, prevent, respond to and recover from all hazards that create health emergencies, including disasters, disease outbreaks and conflicts. This has generated an improved communicable disease surveillance system at the global level, as well as improved national surveillance capacities. Building on the experience of the EVD epidemic in 2014 to 2016 in West Africa, it has also produced a new R&D model for emerging pathogens likely to cause severe outbreaks in the near future, coordinated by the WHO and with the input of a wide range of international scientific and global health agencies (WHO, 2016c). This has already facilitated the development of an effective vaccine against EVD, demonstrating how quickly research can lead to breakthroughs with the right leadership and coordination.

New technologies are enabling scientific breakthroughs in the development of diagnostics, treatment and vaccines for communicable diseases. In late 2016, high-level global initiatives to support the development of new antimicrobial drugs got under way along with new initiatives to fund and fast-track research (Kirby, 2016). Immunization coverage has increased, with an estimated 86% of infants in the world receiving three doses of diphtheria-tetanus-pertussis containing vaccine in 2015 compared with 72% in 2000. Uptake of new and underused vaccines is also increasing (WHO, 2017b). In addition, more people have access to essential health services today than at any other time in history (WHO, 2015). While the number of outbreaks has increased since 1980, research indicates improvements in prevention, early detection, control and treatment mean fewer people have been infected during these outbreaks (Smith *et al.*, 2014).

Summary

In 1962, an eminent scientist said 'to write about infectious diseases is almost to write about something that has passed into history' (Andrewes, 1962). He was not alone in his optimism: the belief that infectious diseases had been successfully overcome was common in biomedical circles at that time (Spellberg and Taylor-Blake, 2013). However, since then it has become clear that such diseases, far from passing into history, continue to be a major threat to human health. New communicable diseases such as HIV and EVD have emerged with devastating consequences. Anthropogenic factors such as climate change, urbanization, land-use change and livestock intensification can increase the emergence of new infectious diseases in humans, and alter the epidemiology and evolution of existing ones. In addition, other well-known diseases, such as malaria and TB, have proven much more difficult to control than anticipated and continue to cause considerable mortality. Poverty and lack of access to essential health services, including vaccination, still result in millions of preventable deaths from communicable disease every year in low-income countries. At the same time, the growth of AMR threatens to render untreatable many infections long considered curable, thus undoing years of medical progress. However, though communicable disease is far from becoming history, there are opportunities for developments and improvements in its control. These include new global initiatives for R&D, improvements in access to vaccination and other essential health services, and improvements in surveillance, control and treatment.

References

Andrewes, C.H. (1962) Book review: Burnet, M. (1962) *Natural History of Infectious Disease*. Cambridge, UK: Cambridge University Press, *British Medical Journal*, 2 (5319): 1588.

Baringer, L. and Heitkamp, S. (2012) Securitizing global health: a view from maternal health, *Global Health Governance*, 4 (2): 1–21.

Centers for Disease Control and Prevention (CDC) (2017) *Emerging Infectious Diseases* journal. Journal background and goals. Available at: https://wwwnc.cdc.gov/eid/page/background-goals [accessed 30 March 2017].

Clarke, T. (2003) Drug companies snub antibiotics as pipeline threatens to run dry, *Nature*, 425 (6955): 225.

Cooper, M. and Shlaes, D.M. (2011) Fix the antibiotic pipeline, *Nature*, 472 (7341): 32.

Curtis, M. (2016) *Gated development: is the Gates Foundation always a force for good?* London: Global Justice Now.

Elbe, S. and Roemer-Mahler, A. (2015) *Global governance and the limits of health security*, IDS Practice Paper in Brief 17. Brighton: Institute of Development Studies. Available at: http://www.ids.ac.uk/publication/global-governance-and-the-limits-of-health-security

European Centre for Disease Prevention and Control (ECDC) (2015) *Infectious diseases of specific relevance to newly arrived migrants in the EU/EEA*, 19 November 2015. Stockholm: ECDC.

Food and Drug Administration (FDA) (2016) *Summary report on antimicrobials sold or distributed for use in food-producing animals*. Available at: https://www.fda.gov/downloads/ForIndustry/UserFees/AnimalDrugUserFeeActADUFA/UCM588085.pdf

Gates, B. (2015) The next epidemic – lessons from Ebola, *New England Journal of Medicine*, 372 (15): 1381–1384.

Gottdenker, N.L., Streicker, D.G., Faust, C.L. and Carroll, C.R. (2014) Anthropogenic land use change and infectious diseases: a review of the evidence, *Ecohealth*, 11 (4): 619–632.

Hawkes, N. (2016) Competition authority will investigate price hikes of generic drugs, *British Medical Journal*, 355: i5849.

Hotez, P.J., Pecoul, B., Rijal, S., Boehme, C., Aksoy, S., Malecela, M. *et al.* (2016) Eliminating the neglected tropical diseases: translational science and new technologies, *PLoS Neglected Tropical Diseases*, 10 (3): e0003895.

Institute for Health Metrics and Evaluation (IHME) (2016) *Financing global health 2015: Development assistance steady on the path to new Global Goals*. Seattle, WA: IHME.

Jones, K.E., Patel, N.G., Levy, M.A., Storeygard, A., Balk, D., Gittleman, J.L. *et al*. (2008) Global trends in emerging infectious diseases, *Nature*, 451 (7181): 990–993.

Kirby, T. (2016) Europe to boost development of new antimicrobial drugs, *The Lancet*, 379 (9833): 2229–2230.

Knobler, S., Mahmoud, A., Lemon, S. and Pray, L. (eds.) (2006) *The Impact of Globalization on Infectious Disease Emergence and Control: Exploring the Consequences and Opportunities: Workshop Summary*. Washington, DC: National Academies Press. Summary and Assessment. Available from: https://www.ncbi.nlm.nih.gov/books/NBK56579/ [accessed 30 March 2017].

McGoey, L. (2015) *No Such Thing as a Free Gift: The Gates Foundation and the Price of Philanthropy*. New York: Verso Books.

Neiderud, C.-J. (2015) How urbanization affects the epidemiology of emerging infectious diseases, *Infection Ecology and Epidemiology*, 5: 10.3402/iee.v5.27060.

New Scientist (2017) Plague! How to prepare for the next pandemic, *New Scientist*, 22 February.

Omran, A.R. (2005) The epidemiologic transition: a theory of the epidemiology of population change, *The Milbank Quarterly*, 83 (4): 731–757.

O'Neill, J. (chair) (2014) *Review on Antimicrobial Resistance – Tackling drug-resistant infections globally* (J. O'Neill, chair). London: HM Government and Wellcome Trust. Available at: https://amr-review. org/sites/default/files/AMR%20Review%20Paper%20-%20Tackling%20a%20crisis%20for%20 the%20health%20and%20wealth%20of%20nations_1.pdf [accessed 30 March 2017].

O'Neill, J. (chair) (2016) *Review on Antimicrobial Resistance. Tackling drug-resistant infections globally: Final report and recommendations* (J. O'Neill, chair). London: HM Government and Wellcome Trust.

Oxford Poverty and Human Development Initiative (OPHI) (2016) *Global multidimensional poverty index 2016*. Available at: http://www.ophi.org.uk/wp-content/uploads/Global-MPI-2016-2-pager.pdf [accessed 6 June 2018].

Ranscombe, P. (2015) The health of nations, *The Lancet Infectious Diseases*, 15 (4): 381.

Saker, L., Lee, K., Cannito, B., Gilmore, A. and Campbell-Lendrum, D. (2004) *Globalization and infectious diseases: A review of the linkages*, Special topics #3. Geneva: UNDP/World Bank/WHO Special Programme on Tropical Diseases Research.

Shuman, E. (2010) Global climate change and infectious diseases, *New England Journal of Medicine*, 362 (12): 1061–1063.

Smith, K.F., Goldberg, M., Rosenthal, S., Carlson, L., Chen, J., Chen. C. *et al*. (2014) Global rise in human infectious disease outbreaks, *Journal of the Royal Society Interface*, 11 (101): 20140950. Available at: http://rsif.royalsocietypublishing.org/content/11/101/20140950 [accessed 30 March 2017].

Spellberg, B. and Taylor-Blake, B. (2013) On the exoneration of Dr. William H. Stewart: debunking an urban legend, *Infectious Diseases of Poverty*, 2 (1): 3.

The Lancet (2009) What has the Gates Foundation done for global health?, *The Lancet*, 373 (9675): 1577.

Udwadia, Z.F., Pinto, L.M. and Uplekar, M.W. (2010) Tuberculosis management by private practitioners in Mumbai, India: has anything changed in two decades?, *PLoS ONE*, 5 (8): e12023.

United Nations Population Fund (UNFPA) (2017) *Migration overview*. Available at: http://www.unfpa. org/migration [accessed 30 March 2017].

United Nations Refugee Agency (UNHCR) (2016) *Figures at a glance*. Available at: http://www.unhcr. org/figures-at-a-glance.html [accessed 30 March 2017].

United Nations Security Council (UNSC) (2014) *Resolution 2177 (2014)*.

United Nations, Department of Economic and Social Affairs, Population Division (UNDESA) (2014) *World urbanization prospects: The 2014 revision*. Available at: https://esa.un.org/unpd/wup/publications/ files/wup2014-report.pdf [accessed 8 June 2018].

Van Boeckel, T.P., Gandra, S., Ashok, A., Caudron, Q., Grenfell, B.T., Levin, S.A. *et al*. (2014) Global antibiotic consumption 2000 to 2010: an analysis of national pharmaceutical sales data, *The Lancet Infectious Diseases*, 14 (8): 742–750.

Van Boeckel, T.P., Brower, C., Gilbert, M., Grenfell, B.T., Levin, S.A., Robinson, T.P. *et al*. (2015) Global trends in antimicrobial use in food animals, *Proceedings of the National Academy of Sciences of the USA*, 112 (18): 5649–5654.

Wirtz, V.J., Hogerzeil, H.V., Gray, A.L., Bigdeli, M., de Joncheere, C.P., Ewen, M.A. *et al*. (2016) Essential medicines for universal health coverage, *The Lancet*, 389 (10067): 403–476.

World Health Organization (WHO) (2007) *World Health Day 2007: International health security*. Available at: http://www.who.int/mediacentre/news/releases/2007/pr11/en/ [accessed 30 March 2017].

World Health Organization (WHO) (2013) *Research priorities for the environment, agriculture and infectious diseases of poverty*, Technical report of the TDR Thematic Reference Group on Environment, Agriculture and Infectious Diseases of Poverty. Geneva: WHO.

World Health Organization (WHO) (2014) *Antimicrobial resistance: Global report on surveillance*. Geneva: WHO. Available at: http://apps.who.int/iris/bitstream/10665/112642/1/9789241564748_eng.pdf [accessed 30 March 2017].

World Health Organization (WHO) (2015) *Tracking universal health coverage: First global monitoring report*. Geneva: WHO. Available at: http://www.who.int/healthinfo/universal_health_coverage/report/2015/en/ [accessed 30 March 2017].

World Health Organization (WHO) (2016a) *Antimicrobial resistance*. Geneva: WHO. Available at: http://www.who.int/mediacentre/factsheets/fs194/en/ [accessed 30 March 2017].

World Health Organization (WHO) (2016b) *World malaria report 2016*. Geneva: WHO. Available at: http://www.who.int/malaria/publications/world-malaria-report-2016/report/en/ [accessed 8 June 2018].

World Health Organization (WHO) (2016c) *An R&D blueprint for action to prevent epidemics*. Geneva: WHO. Available at: http://www.who.int/blueprint/about/r_d_blueprint_plan_of_action.pdf [accessed 8 June 2018].

World Health Organization (WHO) (2017a) *Facts: Urban settings as a social determinant of health*. Available at: http://www.who.int/social_determinants/publications/urbanization/factfile/en/

World Health Organization (WHO) (2017b) *Immunization coverage*, Fact sheet. Available at: http://www.who.int/mediacentre/factsheets/fs378/en/ [accessed 30 March 2017].

Index